MOTIVATION FOR EXERCISE

MOTIVATION FOR EXERCISE

HOW TO GET MOVING AND KEEP MOVING

A PERSONAL GUIDE

Ralph W. Trimble, Ph.D.

ISBN-13: 9781983938351
ISBN-10: 1983938351

CONTENTS

AUTHOR'S NOTE

Throughout the *Guide* I've used stories to illustrate various points or concerns. While they were based on incidents that I've observed or heard about in my working or personal life, I typically changed identifying details or combined several incidents into fictitious amalgamations. Any name I've used, except when referring to my wife or my dad, was chosen at random. Thus while the stories were designed to have broad relevance, any unique resemblance to you, your history, or that of anyone you know, is purely coincidental.

I want to thank the following people for their patient reviews and feedback as I wrote the *Guide*: Robert Sinclair, DDS., my across-the-driveway neighbor and friend, well-known for not holding back on his viewpoints; Paul Joffe, Ph.D., my long-time colleague at the Counseling Center of the University of Illinois and fellow fitness enthusiast; Amy Hassiger, Iowa Writers' Workshop alum, author, teacher and writing consultant; the Red Herring Writers Group at the University of Illinois; and Carolyn Casady Trimble, Ph.D., J.D., fearless critic, tireless supporter, and most importantly, my loving wife.

INTRODUCTION

WHEN I WAS eight, my oldest brother had just graduated from high school, a much acclaimed track star in our hometown of Cedar Rapids, Iowa. He was a state champion in the mile, on his way to a nice athletic scholarship at a Big Ten university. He was my hero. I wanted to follow in his footsteps. As a result, over the next thirteen years, until I graduated from college, motivation for exercise was no problem for me. It was embedded in my desire to perform well in track.

After graduation, performing well in track was no longer a priority. My athletic eligibility at the college level was used up, and I lacked the talent to advance to the next level, running in the pro circuit. It was time for me to pursue another type of career, as a clinical psychologist. I wasn't seeing other reasons to keep exercising.

As I look back, that view seems amazing to me since all along I was getting huge benefits from being fit, benefits well beyond anything to do with track. I knew I felt better and had more energy than most people my age who weren't serious athletes, but I didn't make the connection to fitness. I thought I was just lucky.

Of course I was lucky, but there was more, as I found out after I began graduate school and stopped running. For a few months, I continued to feel great—same free energy, same spring in the legs, and all the rest. Then I began to change. It was as if someone slowly injected thick grease into my system, going beyond lubrication to simply clog things up. I became sluggish and a little cranky, and my concentration was less focused.

My recovery from this funk began when I remembered a conversation I'd had with my dad one evening during my high school years. He'd been an athlete too, a golfer and basketball player. He had fond memories of his days in sports competition, but equally fond memories of how he *felt* when he was so active. These feelings had little to do with winning, team comradery, or sports at all—and a lot to do with fitness and what I was missing now. Recalling his words, I made the connection with fitness, and I started running again—not for track this time, but for quality of life.

I don't want to give the impression that it is always easy to jump into a fitness lifestyle, whether for the first time or after an extended time-off. Depending on your past experiences, it might be easy or it might be hard. My experiences in track made my return fairly easy. Along with my renewed motivation, I'd learned a lot of implementation steps that I needed to turn that motivation into a reality. Thanks to mentoring from my family and from my coaches, I had learned these steps without even realizing that learning was going on. Similarly, I had learned how to structure my thinking and living circumstances so that it was easy to carry out these steps. This learning saved me a lot of sore muscles, unnecessary fatigue and frustration—some of the "costs" that often undermine motivation, causing people to give up.

Fast forwarding my story to the present, I'm seventy-six now, retired from a career as a psychologist at a university counseling center. Throughout the years, I've continued to exercise regularly and receive the perks that go with it. Thanks to an injury I picked up along the way, I don't run any more, but I stay fit by biking, swimming, lifting weights and walking. These activities serve me just as well as running once did, and I'm sure that many other activities could too.

As it turns out, one of our sons, Tom, is a personal trainer in Bellevue, Washington. One of his mottos is "Get fit for life." It's funny how a motto can have multiple meanings, and all of them valid. Initially, I took it to mean, "Get fit and stay that way for the rest of your life," and also, "Get fit so you can do better the things you do in your day-to-day life." But over the years a third meaning has really sunk in: "Get fit so you can enjoy an even better life."

I firmly believe that along with good nutrition, regular exercise is crucial for being "fit for life" in all the ways that I interpret Tom's motto. I won't go so far as to say that regular exercise and good nutrition guarantee you the benefits of fitness, since I still think a certain amount of luck is involved. Not everything is under our control. Going the other way, however, I'm convinced that you won't get all of the perks you're capable of if you don't exercise regularly and practice good nutrition.

Your path toward exercise doesn't have to be the same as mine or anyone else's, and your initial motivations certainly need not involve athletics. Still, as more and more research on exercise-related motivation makes clear, a variety of people who get motivated to exercise and stay motivated have some underlying themes in common.

Among those who neither get nor stay motivated, and who see their fitness levels decline, many share something in common too, namely a tendency to see their lack of motivation as a character flaw, and as something they can never have any control over. I disagree. I see their problem as one of not yet having learned what motivation is, how to get it, how to transform it into exercise and how to keep the motivation and exercise going over the long haul. Motivation for exercise is a learning issue, not a character issue. I've written this *Guide* so you can learn how to develop motivation and then reach a higher quality of life than you might have otherwise.

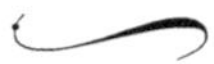

I've written the *Guide* from two perspectives, first, as a clinical psychologist, and second, as a long-time beneficiary of a fitness lifestyle. My formal training, my continued study, and my years of work with clients facing a variety of problems, motivational and otherwise, continually increased my understanding of how how people develop motivation, how they maintain it, and how they turn it into constructive action. Often one of my main tasks was to combine other psychologists' research findings with my clinical experience, and then share that information in ways useful for my clients. That's what I've tried to do with this *Guide,* too.

Early on I learned that the benefits of counseling or therapy are limited if the client only passively participates. A professional can help identify problems, new directions, and ways to move forward, but the client has to be a part of it all and follow through if forward movement is to happen. The same is true for you, the reader. Your active involvement is crucial. To achieve beneficial change, you must think through the approaches, tailor them to your situation, experiment with them, and fine-tune them as your situation changes.

In some ways, as with counseling or therapy, this *Guide* should act as a "springboard," propelling you toward active application. Accordingly, I conclude most chapters with a "Springboard" section, providing suggestions and questions to help you to actively apply the chapter's material to your life.

You may have already learned good approaches for reaching goals in other areas of your life. If you have, the

Guide should help you apply them to achieving a fitness lifestyle. If you haven't, you may find the *Guide's* suggestions for fitness to be useful for those other areas too. Either way, best wishes in developing and maintaining a lifestyle that brings you the many benefits of regular exercise![1]

PART I
OVERVIEW AND BASIC CONCEPTS

C H A P T E R   1

A WARP-SPEED OVERVIEW OF THE *GUIDE*

Motivation and Implementation

FIRST, A WORD about motivation in general, not just exercise-related motivation.[2] Let's start with what motivation is not: Motivation is not a character trait. Rather, motivation is your urge or desire or intention to direct your energy toward a goal-related action or activity.

Imagine you are a high school principal, and nearly every afternoon you are in the middle of conflicts between teachers and parents of adolescents who are allegedly underachieving, misbehaving, victims of overbearing teachers or whatever. You believe that staying calm during these conflicts will boost both your effectiveness and your resistance to burnout. For our purposes, let's have your "goal" be to increase your ability to stay calm. Further, let's suppose that a fellow principal has told you that half-hour walks during her noon-hours help her stay calm during contentious meetings. You're considering whether to have similar walks be a "goal-related" activity for you.

3

To generate motivation for you to take these walks —i.e., to generate a desire or intention to do them—you will need to do two things. First, you must believe that the benefits of walking will outweigh its costs. Second, you must have an expectation that you have a reasonable chance of succeeding in making the walks happen. Let's say you conclude that along with making you more calm, your walks can help you improve your fitness, and that by taking these walks you can set a positive example of self-care for both students and staff. Also, suppose you believe these three "benefits" far outweigh the two "costs" that you envision, namely the price of a pair of walking shoes and the reduced time for eating your lunch. With that belief, you'll have the first prerequisite for motivation. Next, with regard to your "reasonable expectations of success," you already walk your dog for well over a half hour on most Saturdays, so you're confident that your body can handle the effort. Also, thinking of logistics, you reason that having time available at noon is only a matter of having your secretary take your phone calls and protect this time from scheduling, just as he or she does when you have meetings over the noon hour. With the benefits outweighing the costs and with reasonable expectations of being able to carry the activity off, *voila!* You find yourself desiring to walk—you're motivated!

Motivation, though, is only part of the package. You will also need an implementation component to move from desire to action.[3] This includes all of the steps and structuring necessary to insure that your energy gets spent making the goal-relevant activity (in your case, walking) happen, instead of having that energy blocked or diverted elsewhere.

First, your implementation component needs a specific, action-oriented start-up plan. For noon walking, the plan might include things like buying new walking shoes and gradually breaking them in so you don't get blisters, getting into the routine of packing your lunch since you won't have time to eat out, explaining to your secretary why these walks are important so he or she won't feel put upon for having to protect you from interruptions, determining a walking route on the school grounds where students and staff may see your fine example, and making sure the school gym is available for walking during inclement weather. Good start-up plans work like a map, helping you find the right roads and avoid dead ends.

Second, the implementation component needs to include ways to maintain your motivation over the long haul.[4] New challenges arise requiring you to modify even the best of plans. Over time, life has a way of bringing up problems you might not notice or anticipate at first. Some of these you may be able to power through—for a while. For example, when you began your noon walks, maybe packing your own lunch and having to eat it in the limited time left during the noon hour was tolerable, but is starting to become a more irksome cost. Some benefits of exercise that you considered important earlier may come to feel less important later on (for example, keeping calm may be less of an issue as you gain experience with conflicts), or certain costs may seem more important (for example, suppose your boss becomes unhappy with your unavailability during noon hours.)

The barriers requiring maintenance adjustments can seem endless. Maybe you'll encounter distractions that make your plan difficult to follow through on, regardless of its original practicality and regardless of how you feel about the costs and benefits. Changes may alter both your expectations of success and your initial plans—new responsibilities, time drains, energy drains, the impositions of other people's agendas, interruptions, and changes in your physical capabilities that can happen through no fault of your own.

These normal, long-haul challenges require a readiness on your part to respond, rethinking, adjusting, and sometimes simply recovering. None of this has to be rocket science, but it can seem just as difficult at times. Your implementation component is crucial for your motivation's effectiveness and durability. Although I'll sometimes discuss aspects of motivation and implementation separately, they are so intertwined that few discussions in the *Guide* will feature one totally independent of the other, whether or not I refer to them by name.

The remainder of the *Guide* examines in greater depth specifics and life issues of motivation and implementation.

When problems arise it gives you more tools to combat them. The remainder of Part I expands on the specifics of motivation and initial implementation. In Part II, three chapters aim at maximizing your benefits and reducing your costs from exercise, and at increasing your ability to follow through on plans. The five chapters of Part III address long-term challenges to motivation and implementation, increasing your readiness to respond to whatever obstacles you may need to overcome.

C H A P T E R   2

MOTIVATION

Benefits exceeding costs, and expectations of success.

AT THOSE TIMES when you don't understand why you lack motivation to do something, instead of chastising yourself, stop and re-evaluate. You may not be considering all of your feelings about the activity's related costs and benefits. Also, you may be ignoring (low) expectations of success with the activity. Motivation has two key requirements: (1) you must believe that the benefits of doing something outweigh its costs, and (2) you must expect a reasonable chance of success in attempting it. If on re-examination, the benefits seem too small or the costs seem too big, or if you aren't seeing a strong likelihood of success, your motivation will undoubtedly falter.

All of this may be hard to really understand without examples. Let's begin with a couple of very unlikely ones from the world of sports and then consider several others perhaps closer to home.

Picture Joe, a highly talented college basketball player, one whom all the NBA scouts want to draft because they think he can become the next superstar. The only catch

8

is that while Joe likes basketball and has had a lot of fun playing most of his life, for him the thrill is gone. Instead, his big dream now is to become a high-powered business executive. Joe is very bright, he's gotten a great education, and he comes from a wealthy family with lots of connections in the business world, so his business dreams are not far-fetched. On the other hand, the only things a pro-basketball career represent to Joe are a now meaningless activity, too much time away from his fiancé, and a delay in starting his "real" career. He will have plenty of money either way. Thus, he thinks that at graduation it will be time for him to stop playing basketball and instead to follow his real dream.

Despite the fact that Joe has motivation's second crucial ingredient—very reasonable expectations for success in the NBA—he clearly does not believe the benefits of a pro-basketball career outweigh the costs. As a result, he is not motivated to enter the draft, much less play pro ball. Now, let's reverse the strengths of these ingredients:

Suppose, in contrast to Joe, I—of all people—were to really want to play basketball in the NBA. Suppose I would enjoy every aspect of that life—the workouts, the competition, the travel, the adulation, the money, and—on the other side—even the hectic, endless season of body pounding and time away from family. Clearly I would have the first crucial ingredient, the benefits outweighing the costs. However, only if I were delusional to the point of being psychotic would I carry any expectation of success. I'm old, I'm short, and even when I was young I was a lousy basketball player.

I would lack the necessary expectations of success. Neither Joe nor I would want to direct our energies toward getting into the NBA; neither of us would be motivated.

Craig's problems are much more typical: After heart surgery, his cardiologist put him on a walking program, hoping to prevent a future cardiac crisis. Craig stayed with the program for several months. Unfortunately, over time, he started skipping his walks for various reasons, and eventually stopped the program altogether. For better or worse (and his cardiologist worries about the latter) he feels fine right now, and his concerns over a future crisis seem less important as the months go along. As he explains, he can't overcome other concerns like the boredom he feels when he's on the treadmill or the time that walking outside takes from his other activities. Of course, if you pinned him down, he would tell you that staying alive is more important than these other things, but on a daily basis, when it is time to walk, these other concerns occupy more of the picture for him.

Craig's motivational problems involve the costs and benefits he sees and feels on a daily basis. Chapter Four suggests a number of ways to increase motivation by increasing the benefits, and Chapter Five suggests a number of ways to reduce costs. Meanwhile, other remedies for Craig could include modifying the type of exercise and the places he exercises. He could also systematically and frequently re-evaluate *all* of his priorities.

Jenny's problem involves costs and benefits too: When Jenny was single, she had a membership at a fitness center which she used nearly every day. She loved the feeling of exhilaration that her workouts gave her. Now she is married to Hank, they have a baby, and they feel reluctant to trust the baby to a sitter. Hank jogs before Jenny and their baby get up, and says he wouldn't mind watching their baby later so she could go to the gym. Unfortunately, the guilt she would feel "dumping" the baby on Hank while she's off "having fun" keeps Jenny at home.

Jenny's motivational problem comes from costs—feelings of guilt—outweighing benefits. Assuming Hank really means it when he says he's willing to baby-sit, Jenny's guilt may stem from many other things. Let's assume her guilt stems from her misinterpreting Hank's feelings. Previous misunderstandings with Hank might be making her unduly hesitant to take his words at face value. If so, it might help if Jenny and Hank worked on communication problems with the aid of a trained professional.

Mike's problems are more with his expectations of success: Mike would love to become more fit, and for him, a single guy with a good job, common issues like time, inconvenience, money or family concerns are minimal. The sticking point for Mike is his own history of failure with any physical endeavor. As a child, Mike was overweight and clumsy. His peers laughed at him in gym class. Now, although his peers have grown up enough to not laugh at him anymore, he still lacks confidence when attempting anything physical. He feels a sense of hopelessness and pessimism. "I've always been an overweight klutz and I always will be, so why beat a dead horse?"

Mike might consider entering the world of exercise with activities he already can do, such as walking. Regular walking could bring multiple rewards if he gave it a chance. Beginning with the level of demand quite low, and only gradually increasing it, his initial goals wouldn't have to depend on a backlog of skill or stamina. Regardless of Mike's background—or yours—motivation requires realistic demands and expectations.

Andrea has expectations problems too, but from a different direction: When Andrea was in high school, she was active in team sports. She always got into shape quickly, and if she got injured, she healed quickly. Then after twenty years spent focusing on other important things, such as her job and her family, she found herself overweight and feeling slowed down. She decided to start an exercise program at a nearby gym.

Many people have regained their fitness after years of inactivity, but not with the overly optimistic expectations that Andrea carried into the effort—expectations based on her high school experiences. She overlooked the fact that she was now approaching forty. She underestimated how long it would take to rebuild her endurance, lose extra pounds, and heal from the exercise-related soreness and injuries she suffered along the way.

Over the next two years, Andrea began several exercise programs full blast, repeatedly challenging her body at her high school speed. Repeatedly her body rebelled and she experienced excessive fatigue and injuries. Friends told her to take things more slowly and gradually, but she refused. She'd say, "What good would that do?" or "Anyone can do that!" Unfortunately, this approach took its toll on her body and her motivation. Now Andrea's expectations have gone to the opposite extreme, and she doesn't exercise at all, simply saying, "Hey, I'm too old for this stuff! I know when I'm licked!"

Some helpful changes for Andrea could include combining low-impact group exercise such as water aerobics, zumba or tai chi (she liked team sports in high school) with explanations from a personal trainer about the importance and meaningfulness of slower, more gradual increases in fitness over time.

I want to emphasize that in none of these cases have I made any references to character, guts, IQ or any negative personal judgment. Neither judgmental concepts nor personality makeovers nor brain transplants are the answer. Solutions for motivational problems come from finding ways to improve the benefit-cost ratios and to realistically improve the expectations of success.

Individual Tailoring: Putting yourself into the story.
Of course, all the above examples are simplified. Real-life motivational problems are rarely a matter of only a few cost-benefit issues or only a few expectations. Most of the time motivation actually involves an intermingling of both types of issues, and many of the factors are more subtle. At least, that's the way it is when you or I have motivational problems. Right?

Because motivational problems, like people, are highly individual, the solutions will be unique to each person. This book can't provide THE solution for your specific case. But it can give you tools and ideas to try out and incorporate, as you personally tailor a motivational solution that works for you.

These tools and ideas will help you structure your exercise program in a way that always gives you benefits, both immediate and long-term, which outweigh the costs you are likely to feel along the way. They can also help you structure your program in a way that some success is always a reasonable and interesting thing to expect, whether at your beginning level or at higher levels later on.

Springboard.
In Chapter Three, I'll be encouraging you to design and implement an initial exercise program where you take the motivational concerns of this chapter seriously. Before going there, however, I hope you'll give some thought to the following questions. You'll get more out

of the questions if you write down your answers, coming back to them from time to time, and adding new thoughts as they occur to you:

1. What are the possible benefits of a fitness lifestyle for you personally?[5]
   -- Benefits can include a wide variety of positive consequences, things you would like. What positive benefits would you like to receive through a fitness lifestyle?
   -- Benefits can also include the escape or avoidance of some negative consequences, things you dislike. What negative consequence(s) would you like to escape or avoid through a fitness lifestyle?
2. What about your possible costs in seeking a fitness lifestyle?
   -- Costs can include a variety of discomforts, both physical and emotional. What discomforts would you experience with a fitness lifestyle?
   -- Costs can also include losses, things you would have to give up. What losses would a fitness lifestyle entail?
   -- Costs can also include conflicts and/or inconveniences for you or for people you care about. What conflicts or inconveniences are likely to result for yourself or other people if you adopted a fitness lifestyle?

[If you have not already chosen the type of exercise you want to do, postpone work on the next item (#3) until finishing the Springboard for Chapter Three.]

3. What are your hopes and expectations for success in achieving a fitness lifestyle? Central to the success of most approaches is the identification of an exercise demand level which is comfortable now, with the idea of perhaps gradually increasing that demand over time, but NEVER out-pacing your readiness. That allows you to continually succeed without having the demands get so high that your costs outweigh your benefits. Your development of fitness doesn't happen overnight. There's no quick fix.

   [Hint: If a current demand level is so high that you are tired for the rest of the day, you've set it too high. Along with lowering the demand, you also may need to allow some recovery time before resuming. Also, some muscle soreness is likely at first. To prevent that soreness from turning into an injury, allow adequate recovery time for that too.]

Don't be discouraged if you don't have answers to some of these questions. You can always come back and put in answers or change your initial ones in light of later chapters and your exercise experiences along the way.

CHAPTER 3

IMPLEMENTATION

Turning Your Intentions into Actions

WHEN YOU SAY you feel motivated to start a fitness program, very likely you mean something like you "want" or "intend" to start exercising on a regular basis. You may be feeling energized, and certainly you're thinking that being fit is desirable. Often it feels good to be motivated. That's fortunate, because motivation is a key factor in having a lasting program. However, much research over the last three decades has made it clear that while motivation is necessary, it's not sufficient. You also need an implementation component to provide steps, processes and structures for transforming the intentions and energy of your motivation into action.

Motivation answers the "why" question: "Why do I want to improve my fitness?" For motivated people, the various answers tend to boil down to something like, "Because fitness has a huge pay-off and I'm capable of having it!" The implementation component answers the "how" question, "How am I going to make my fitness program happen and keep happening?"

Two major parts of a good implementation component are Initial Plans and Maintenance Adjustments. As the names imply, your Initial Plans emphasize the steps and structures you will follow to get the fitness program started and your Maintenance Adjustments emphasize the changes you must make over time to keep the program going. Initial Plans address such questions as:

What activities are you going to do? Suppose you want something aerobic, but you hate to swim and your knees can't tolerate the impact of jogging. For purpose of illustration, let's say you choose biking.

Where will you exercise? Do you have easy access to bike paths or small, lightly used, hard-surface country roads?

With or without other people? Your choice, certainly, but in starting, you might want to bike alone so you don't have to worry about slowing your friends down.

When? During daylight hours, of course, and at times of light traffic, but also take into account possible schedule conflicts for both you and your significant others.

How often? Especially at first, perhaps every other day, since your body requires more recovery time for new activities. On your off days consider an easy walk to stimulate circulation and loosen up.

How demanding or intense? Again, especially at first, err on the conservative side, both in duration and intensity. Increase gradually, and never have the demands you put on yourself exceed your then-current abilities.

In making your plans, stack the cards so the benefits clearly outweigh the costs. Weigh all the benefits, mental as well as physical. For example, the bonus benefits of biking can include enjoying the scenery along the way or a temporary escape from other people's demands.

While setting up your Initial Plans, start thinking about Maintenance Adjustments, the changes you will have to make as needed to keep the program going. You and your circumstances will change over time. If you don't adjust, your fitness programs and your motivation will fade away. In the biking example above, even during Initial Planning, it wouldn't be too soon to start thinking of what adjustments you'll make for bitterly cold weather—some people put their bikes on wind trainers and "bike" indoors while watching movies or TV. Others, in milder climates, simply buy warmer clothing for continued outdoor biking.

For the *Guide* I've divided Maintenance Adjustment concerns into two sections. One section, Part II, relates to the fundamental concepts of Costs, Benefits and Initial Plans. The other, Part III, addresses some of what may be termed "life's challenges." Addressing all the possible obstacles you might encounter is beyond the scope of the *Guide,* so my goal has been to cover enough to guide you on how to react successfully if additional obstacles pop up. Meanwhile, let's go back to making Initial Plans and trying out a first exercise program.

Getting started.

If you don't already have an exercise program, I urge you to begin one now. You may think that I haven't told you enough for you to do that yet—and, in a way, I agree. You shouldn't expect your first effort to be a lasting program. If you are like most people, your motivation will begin to trail off soon after you've started your new program, and you'll find yourself skipping your exercise for reasons that don't seem valid when you review them later on. This is normal.

You need some trial-and-error experience and you need more information. The trouble is that you won't know which information you'll need—and it may be hard to have a feel for it—until you've tried a few things out. The goal, then, is not to have you come up with a lasting program on your first attempt. However, I hope that your initial attempt will get you used incorporating the concepts of benefits, costs, and expectations of success as you plan. You should also get used to thinking in terms of steps and structures which will help you achieve your fitness goals. And finally, your experiences in this first start should accelerate your ability to make good uses of Parts II and III on your next attempt.

As you plan and try out your first program, pay attention to what helps or hinders your motivation and your progress. For example, suppose walking is your exercise. If you want to walk after work, are you able to leave your office early enough to walk before you have to pick up your children or get home for dinner? Being able to do that will certainly help your motivation and your progress. Suppose you decide that the noon hour is your best time to walk: Do you have trouble saying "No" to your co-workers when they want you to join them for lunch? Do you typically schedule work-related meetings then? Such conflicts may lower your motivation. Do you enjoy encouraging others to walk with you? That might actually help you. On the other hand, do you hate to sweat? If so, can you accommodate that in some way or is it a "deal breaker?"

Sometimes you won't be able to recognize what helps or hinders you until you notice that it comes up repeatedly as a pattern. A pattern is a sequence of events that seem to go together time after time, so that you find yourself saying, "Whenever X happens, it seems as if I end up doing Y." For example, you may find yourself saying, "Whenever it's raining in the morning, I end up sleeping late instead of taking a jog." Seeing the pattern can give you clues to the remedy—such as setting up a place to come inside while wet without making a mess or buying a rain suit. In the spirit of this example and the earlier one of biking inside on a wind trainer during cold weather, remember the saying, "No bad weather, just bad equipment!"

Again, it's not important that your first exercise program works very well. The important thing is that it provides you with the basis for some self-assessment and identifications of problems you'll want to fix in your next program. Before trying your initial program you won't know which obstacles and patterns may interfere. What you learn will help you make your next set of plans more effective, as well as help you get more out of Parts II and III.

Springboard.
Here are some helpful suggestions for getting started:

1. To choose the type of exercise you'll be doing:
    a. Write down what benefits you most want.
    b. List all of the types of activities that you think might provide these benefits. Consult with your physician, with a personal trainer, and/ or withfriends for ideas, recommendations, and cautions. Proceed with legitimate assurance that what you are doing will be safe for you.
    c. List the likely costs for each of these activities.
    d. Eliminate any exercise option where it seems obvious that the costs will be too big or the benefits too small.
    e. Further, concerning expectations, eliminate any option where it seems obvious that your chances of following it successfully are low.
    f. Choose among the remaining alternatives on the basis of your personal likes and dislikes.

g. Finally, decide where you will exercise, whether with or without supervision, when, and how often.

2. Organize your activity so that each time you do it, the immediate benefits you feel (such as enjoyments, satisfactions or feelings of accomplishment) outweigh any of its costs (such as inconvenience or fatigue). You may find that keeping a daily workout log helps you make a fair assessment of ongoing costs and benefits as well as monitor your progress. For example, suppose during today's morning walk you were unusually effective in anticipating and thinking through a challenge you had to face later in the day. Maybe the relaxed setting of the walk was just what you needed for this kind of thinking. If so, "celebrate" by commenting on the experience in your workout log.

3. Address the issue of reasonable expectations:

a. Injuries lower your chances of success. You can prevent many injuries by consulting with professionals on such things as proper equipment (including running or walking shoes), and proper technique (especially if you do any weight lifting).

b. Always seek a level of difficulty you can "master," either presently or soon. Such mastery not only is rewarding in itself but is likely to be your most important basis for expecting success at the next level.[6]

c. At the beginning of any next level, if you are not sure how much to challenge yourself, err on the light side and see how you feel over the next few days. If you find yourself unduly tired or sore, go lighter still until your body starts to adjust. This is good for injury prevention as well as for motivation.

d. Only after your body seems to have adjusted should you gradually increase the challenges.

e. Don't worry if your increases in activity are slower or smaller than someone else's. Another person's more rapid increases in activity may contribute to their quitting later on. You aren't in a contest or up against a deadline. Rather, you're working on a long-term process. As the tortoise observed, "Slow and steady wins the race."

4. Give this first program a fair try. That includes not only doing it, but trying to stick with it for two to five weeks.[7]

5. As you go along, notice your physical and emotional reactions. Again, keeping a log can help you. Be a detective! Take note of variations in your motivation and variations in your adherence to the routine. When you notice these variations, ask yourself whether anything else might be going

on that's related to them. Look for patterns and discover what helps or hinders your motivation.

You may set up this first program and stay with it forever. More likely, though, you'll find your motivation and workout routine deteriorate after several weeks. Rather than viewing that as bad news, consider it a necessary reality check. Now you'll have had experiences that will help you make better plans and better uses of Parts II and III of the *Guide.*

Oh! By the way: If you are one of the lucky few for whom Part I was enough to help you get on track and keep on track, that's great! You'll have gotten what you need without having to read the rest of the *Guide,* and you can give your copy to a friend.

PART II

ADDING MUSCLE TO YOUR COST/ BENEFIT RATIO AND TO YOUR PLANS

CHAPTER 4

INCREASING YOUR BENEFITS

The Problem: The benefits you seek might not be enough by themselves.
Often people want to get fit so they will be healthier, more attractive or more proficient in a sport. Perhaps they want to play basketball or tennis with their colleagues or they want to walk along the paths of Italy's Cinque Terre. Maybe they want to run, or at least walk, a 5K or even a half-marathon. There is certainly nothing wrong with any of these benefits, but by themselves they may fail to keep a person motivated long enough to make the desired differences. There are lots of reasons why. Do any of these sound familiar?

The desired benefit doesn't always seem to link clearly enough to the fitness activity. For example, after several months, a person may say, "I've not had that second heart attack yet, but how do I know if it was because of my diet and exercise?"

After a while the benefit may seem less important. In effect, a person may say, "You know, most of the time I don't really care that much if I'm a few pounds too heavy. I'm happy and my friends like me just the way I am."

The benefit doesn't always come consistently enough. A person might say, "I made steady improvements at first, but not as much lately."

The delay between the effort and the resulting benefit may seem too long. For example, a would-be runner might say, "Sure, I'd love to be in a 10K road race, but it would take forever to get in shape for it."

SOLUTIONS

You can increase the motivational impact of any fitness-related benefit in three major ways: first, with validation; second, through ownership of the fitness program; and third, by regulating the program's difficulty level. In addition, I'll suggest some easy ways for you to increase the number of auxiliary benefits beyond those you might have originally had in mind. And finally, I'll emphasize putting your daily focus on achieving positive outcomes, even if your more important goal is to avoid a negative outcome, such as a heart attack.

Increasing the impact of the benefits through validation.
A Sunday comic strip once showed Calvin and Hobbs sliding down a steep, snow-covered hill on their toboggan. As they sped along, Calvin got philosophical. He noted that sliding like this was "OK," but to make it really good, it would need to be filmed and documented on a TV show like "Sixty Minutes." In other words, sliding

wasn't really good unless it got attention, adulation and—most basically—validation from other people. Like many good jokes, the humor came from identifying a common human need and then exaggerating it. In this case, most of us like to have others' validation of the things we do.[8]

As long as the need isn't so strong that it totally runs your life, there is nothing wrong with it. More positively, others can help you make better decisions about your fitness habits and help you keep up your motivation. In the case of fitness activities, another person's support can weaken the effects of those rationalizations any of us can fall into, where we justify eating the second dessert or skipping today's workout. Also, a friend's support can help make doing the workout feel worthwhile. Consider the case of Patty.

Patty liked her water aerobics class. It met three times a week (M, W, F) at 6 a.m., and there was another slightly different class she could attend two other days (T, Th). The exercise was helping her trim down, but still she was starting to waver in her motivation. She had no validation at all from friends. Some of her friends were indifferent and others thought water aerobics classes were a waste of time. While she valued these people in other ways and wanted to keep them as friends, she realized that she needed to surround herself with additional friends to help her keep going. One day after water aerobics class, she initiated having breakfast with several of her classmates. Also, at work, she began to talk about the class with several people. By reaching out in such ways, she soon learned that there were many people around her who thought it was great that she was trying to keep fit. Their encouragement helped her continue to value exercise, and she gained—rather than lost—friends in the process.

Increasing the impact of benefits through ownership.
All of us can use help in keeping the importance of good nutrition and exercise in mind. The support and encouragement of friends can be one good source of help with implementing changes and improvements in our routines. On the other hand, relying on such support and encouragement can be overdone and become harmful. The reason for this has to do with a quiet, but steady, drive within each of us to seek personal ownership and control over our actions. Other people and the incentives they may offer (such as praise, criticism, money or deprivations) may cause you to put this drive on hold for a while, but eventually the value you place on an activity will lessen if you do not feel a personal sense of ownership and control over it. Eventually, you may become indifferent to the activity itself or feel rebellious toward it or toward the well-intended people who are pushing you to do it.

Courtney's experience is a case in point: Courtney and Bob had been married for several years when Courtney realized that she had put on some weight. Bob had never criticized or even mentioned her weight gain, and didn't seem particularly upset by it, but when she decided to make some changes, he took it upon himself to be her full-fledged supporter—and then some.

Bob went with Courtney when she consulted a personal trainer and a nutritionist, he took copious notes during both visits, and he assumed most of the responsibility for fine-tuning "the program" when they got home. This included setting up exercise and diet charts and buying a scale. Then, each morning he reminded her of what "the program" called for that day. Each evening he checked off the various items on the charts. And each Sunday morning, he weighed her (!).

Before long, Courtney's motivation began to lag, and Bob reacted with more vigorous encouragement. Not long after that, Courtney refused to continue "the program" and they began fighting over many things having nothing to do with fitness.

Their next consultation was with a marriage counselor, after which their relationship got back on track. Eventually Courtney got back on a fitness program—her program. This time Bob kept totally out of it, and everything went a lot better for each of them.

Courtney's turn-around became possible because eventually she and Bob were able to talk about the problem and give the ownership and control to her. After that, Courtney was able to enjoy the benefits of fitness activities and keep her motivation high.

Increasing the impact by regulating the program's difficulty level. Whatever the fitness activity, if it is too easy, you may not feel as if you've accomplished much after you have finished it. That can be true even if the activity is somewhat enjoyable. On the other hand, if you make that same activity impossibly hard, you may not feel much accomplishment either. Instead, you'll simply feel overwhelmed.

Fortunately, you can select an "optimal" level of difficulty or challenge, one between these extremes. Your optimal level should be where the activity is possible for you to do, but not ridiculously easily. Indeed, it should take you a reasonable amount of effort, but not so much that you are feeling especially tired or sore the next day. By working at an optimal level, you'll have the satisfaction of accomplishing something. Equally important, you won't feel punished and hesitant to put in the necessary amount of effort again next time. Obviously, when you feel as if you've accomplished something, the experienced value of your exercise will be higher and you'll feel more motivated.

Randy wanted to get in shape to run with his partner, Kim, who frequently ran in 5K road races. He had never run with a race in mind, and he was concerned that he might look bad compared to her. She advised him to start out gradually, first with long walks. Kim also suggested that after several weeks of walking he gradually introduce block-long intervals of slow jogging into the walks; from there she suggested that he gradually lengthen the jogging intervals; and after that, gradually increase the speed. Finally, she said, after four or five months, they could workout together, doing the workouts she was already doing. Eventually they could run in some 5Ks together.

Randy found this advice to be a bit condescending. After a week of easy walks where he came back feeling as if he'd done nothing while Kim came back from her run flushed and exhilarated, he declared it was time to increase his difficulty level.

Unfortunately, he went too far. The next day, against her advice, Randy insisted on running Kim's workout with her. It happened that she was doing a four-mile run; he almost made two of the four miles before he was exhausted and slightly nauseated. He felt miserable for the rest of the day, he had blisters on both heels, and after a bad night of sleep he was so sore that he could barely get out of bed.

Following that experience, Randy revised his program yet again. This time, he began with two weeks of short intervals of slow jogging during long walks. Each week after that, he gradually increased the difficulty level, usually in terms of interval distance but sometimes in terms of speed. The daily goals always required enough effort so that he felt as if he was accomplishing something, and he had a feeling of fun and satisfaction in the process. Three months later, he and Kim were working out together on many days, and five months later he and Kim ran in their first 5K together.

Perhaps like many of us, Randy was hampered initially by some misplaced competitive concerns and a macho hang-up or two. Be that as it may, after his negative experience he put his focus on setting a goal at the optimal level for each day, and things worked out much better.

Two other points from Randy's experience are worth noting: First, it's not always easy to know what your optimal level of difficulty is, so you may have to go through some trial and error before you find it. Second, as Randy got into better shape, his optimal level of difficulty rose. By the time he was running 5Ks with Kim, even much of his revised plan would have felt too easy to be meaningful.

Choosing activities and approaches that give additional benefits. Even with a sense of ownership, with validation from others, and with the level of activity well regulated, a benefit can start to feel inadequate by itself. Part of the solution can come from choosing an activity that helps you achieve other goals as well as the ones related to health, attractiveness or performance enhancement.

Consider Libby's case: On her annual medical exam, Libby's doctor warned her that her blood pressure and cholesterol were elevated. She didn't like the idea of medications for the rest of her life. Fortunately, the doctor gave her three months to try getting them under control without drugs. He strongly encouraged Libby to get on an exercise program and to reduce her daily caloric intake. Unfortunately, he gave her no guidance about how to implement his suggestions. She was on her own.

Libby tried to follow her doctor's orders—first with swimming and then with walking on a treadmill—and each time gave up after several weeks. Both times she noticed that on days when she exercised, she had less difficulty limiting her caloric intake, but exercise and calorie control took a back seat whenever anything else came up in her busy life.

Not surprisingly, Libby found herself dreading seeing her doctor for her three-month check. She shared her concern with a friend who suggested that she get that dog she had always wanted. He knew Libby would be conscientious about giving a dog daily walks, regardless of what she would do otherwise for herself when feeling rushed.

Libby liked the idea—it was just the additional reason she needed to get a dog anyway. She chose a puppy from a breed that that was easily trained and would like long walks, and she followed through. She trained the dog to walk by her side, not pulling on the lead (which would have hurt her shoulder or back), so that walks were pleasant for both of them. When that dog died, a number of years later, she got another. Over those years, her cholesterol and blood pressure returned to the normal ranges and stayed there, she had fun with her dogs, and she found that the errands and other activities that used to pre-empt a fitness lifestyle either got done anyway or didn't need to be done in the first place.

Libby is not the only one who has achieved additional benefits from her exercise program. George, with the help of a personal trainer, designed a weight lifting and stair master program that not only made him look more buff but also prepared him for a week of wilderness canoeing, portaging and camping with his son the following summer. Alice took up yoga, not just for her arthritis, but also so she could get down on the floor and play with her grandchildren. John, an air traffic controller, realized that exercise gave him a daily mini-vacation from stress as well as a flatter stomach. And on and on . . . .

We live in an outcome-oriented society, but along with outcome benefits, it is important to cultivate process benefits. Outcome benefits usually come after doing an activity over an extended period of time—for example, increased stamina after several months of biking. On the other hand, process benefits come during the workout or soon thereafter, and are more temporary. You can usually feel a reduction in stress after ten or fifteen minutes into a workout. It's a benefit that won't last forever. You'll need to work for it day by day. But it is still good.

Design your program with both outcome and process orientations in mind. Look at it this way: you probably started your fitness program to get a certain outcome, for example, weight loss. If the only thing you focus on is that long-term benefit, you'll have to go through long dry spells, plateaus where no weight loss occurs, but with lots of time to develop doubts, get distracted, or simply shove some of your initial concerns out of your mind. If you have a process orientation as well as an outcome orientation, those plateaus won't be so dry because you'll be getting some benefits (process benefits) each day— and you'll more likely ride the plateau through and ultimately reach your (outcome) goal.

Ask yourself what felt good about today's workout. Only the shower? Well, perhaps you need to reduce the intensity of the workout or get more sleep, but in the meantime, make it a point to at least enjoy that shower! Did you see anyone interesting or hear anything interesting today at the gym? Were any of the exercises fun today? If not, did you nevertheless get a feeling of satisfaction from doing some of them? (Having "fun" is not always a prerequisite for feeling satisfaction.) Did you achieve any sub-goal today? That's great! Congratulate yourself! Even when you are making good progress overall, you'll have plateaus and minor setbacks, so each sub-goal is something to celebrate. (See below regarding sub-goals.)

All of these "process questions" carry a clear implication concerning your mindset. With the outcome orientation you focus on only one or two dimensions (such as weight loss). With the process orientation, you stay aware of a number of dimensions. Along with attention to your sub-goals (such as one pound lost per week), you stay aware of your senses, of other people, and of anything interesting that may be going on while you're working out. Tunnel vision, where you look only at the end, ignoring everything to the sides, is fine for some endeavors, but may not be enough for maintaining long-term fitness motivation. Some people prefer to cling to tunnel vision for fear they will stray from the course they have set. If that describes you, as long as your process benefits are compatible with your workout plan, this isn't necessarily a problem. You may need a narrow focus for some parts of your day, but here, during exercise time, it can be good to open your mind.

Here's one more important process point: The daily workout becomes an emotional mini-vacation from the rest of the day for many people. You don't have to forbid your office problems from coming into your mind during the workout, but when you're breathing hard, maybe you'll feel less concerned about them than you did a half an hour earlier. And in contrast to that half-hour earlier, maybe right now you can open up to a few other things going on around you. The office problems will still be there when you get back to them, but they will hit you with less emotional punch if the workout helped you see a bigger picture. In effect, the bigger picture can tell you that your office problems aren't the only things going on in your world right now, and that you'll survive, even if the office really is in trouble. And sometimes the mini-vacation can help you open your mind to a solution for whatever problem was bothering you back at the office.

Actually, some people will tell you that the main benefits they seek from exercise *are* process benefits: "I exercise and eat right because doing so makes me feel better at the time as well as later." Of course, while they continue to feel better, they also look better and enjoy good health, but for them these are side benefits.

Sub-goals can provide a link between your process orientation and your outcome orientation; they are the stair steps between where you are now and the place you want to reach. If you want go three floors up from where you are now, you certainly won't get there in a couple of steps, much less in a single bound, like Superman. Clearly you'll need to take a lot of smaller steps. Sometimes in your planning you'll find that you've made some of the steps too easy and others too hard. You can re-adjust difficulty level, but having set steps gives you some present (that is, process) indication of whether you are moving toward your overall goal. When you find yourself progressing, you get a motivational boost. In contrast, when you find yourself slipping, you may need to ask what else is going on to cause the problem. Is it due to making the steps too large? Falling behind on your rest? Stresses in other parts of your life?

Beyond the answers to such questions, remember that you won't see progress on an outcome dimension every day anyway—progress graphs are often saw-tooth affairs with only the over-all trends looking right. On some days your only discernable benefits may be just your process benefits. Notice them and don't take them for granted.

My next suggestion follows directly from the common observation that even in our culture, where achieving tangible objectives is often used as a measure of success, people still can get personal satisfaction from developing skills, from gaining "mastery" over what they do and from gaining knowledge about themselves and the world. This satisfaction is available when you step back and pay attention to something other than the external incentives and pressures in your life. Try adding skill goals and knowledge goals to the various performance goals or outcome goals you already have in your fitness program.

For example, if you are swimming, take some swim lessons, improve your favorite stroke, learn some new strokes, or learn how to do flip turns. If you are weight lifting, hire a personal trainer to show you the proper movements—techniques and exercises that will not only help you get stronger but also help you avoid injuries. If you are running, read up on what the experts advise for safely improving your sprinting speed. If you're a walker, learn about proper form and posture, and perhaps also learn something about the architecture or history of the neighborhoods you pass through or the types of flowers or birds you see along the way.

My wife, Carolyn, who has walked and run in our neighborhood for over forty years, knows where the most beautiful trees and bushes are for each season. She recognizes the songs of various migrating birds as they pass through in the spring and fall. And the gardens along her route give her ideas of what to plant next year in our yard. The enjoyment and satisfaction you get from pursuing "skill goals" and "knowledge goals" will add to the benefits of your fitness lifestyle and help you keep your motivation high.

Focusing on "positive" benefits more than on "negative" benefits.[9] A positive benefit is something that you want to make happen and that you think of as good. A negative benefit involves preventing something bad from happening. An example of a negative benefit of a fitness program might be preventing a heart attack. Obviously your negative benefit can be more important than any positive benefit on the horizon. Unfortunately, it is also difficult to tell whether you've really achieved it. Thus in general, even when doing exercises to obtain an important negative benefit, you'll get more motivational mileage by putting most of your daily focus on the interim and positive benefits.

In contrast to the negative benefit, positive benefits are more pleasant to focus on, especially over an extended time. More importantly, your efforts to follow through, if aiming at positive benefits, are likely to be more stable and less open-ended than if you only aim at the negative benefits. Usually your progress toward the positive benefits will be more immediately tangible. You can easily tell when you start being able to walk comfortably for twenty minutes, or feel good enough to play on the floor with your grandchild. But how do you know whether your exercising is moving you away from a heart attack? Check-ups with your cardiologist help, but you can't just drop in each day after workout to see if you're safer now. The lack of this sort of feedback during the intervals between check-ups can feel like long, dry spells. It can strain your motivation.

If you select your positive benefits carefully and focus on them when they happen, you can be far less reliant on imagination for motivational power than would be the case with focus only on negative benefits. Again, positive benefits may not be as important as, say, preventing a heart attack, but focusing on them can aid your prevention efforts and do so in ways that help make your continuing life more worthwhile.

Springboard.
To more easily increase the benefits of a fitness program, and to optimize their impact on your motivation, answer the following questions. As always, it's useful to write your answers down and come back to them from time to time for further thought:

1. Validation,
    a. Who currently supports your fitness activities?
    b. Do you need more support from these or other people?

    ___ No ___ Yes If yes, with whom might you generate more support, and how?

2. Ownership: Friends and professionals may encourage you, but for the benefits to keep on having their full impact, you must have a personal sense of ownership and control over your fitness activities. Do you?

    ___ Yes ___ No If no, how might you constructively regain ownership? (Here see the section on Assertive Communication in Chapter Ten.)

3. Optimal level of difficulty: Does your fitness program seem either too easy or too hard?

    ___ No ___ Yes If yes, how might you raise or lower the difficulty level a few steps?

4. Multiple benefits and goals: Beyond your initial reasons for getting fit, are there additional benefits or goals that a different activity or a modification of your present activity could help you achieve?

    ___ No ___ Yes If yes,

    a. What are the additional benefits or goals?

    b. What changes would you need to make?

5. Process benefits: Beyond the long-range outcome benefits of your fitness program,

    a. What are some possible process benefits you might start tuning in to?

    b. What could be your first steps?

6. Skill and knowledge goals:

    a. What aspects of your fitness routine might be fun to learn more about or get better at?

    b. What would be your first steps?

7. Putting most of your focus on positive benefits:

    a. Is a negative benefit your main reason for fitness activity?

    ___ No ___ Yes If yes, what is it?

    b. Do you get any positive benefits from your fitness activity?

___ No ___ Yes If yes, what are they? If no, how might you start having some positive benefits?

    c. As you follow your fitness program, do you give more attention to positive or to negative benefits?

___ Positive ___ Negative If you attend more to negative than to positive benefits, how can you increase the number of positive benefits, or at least increase your attention to the positive benefits already available?

CHAPTER 5

REDUCING YOUR COSTS

The Problem: Benefits must exceed costs.

In Chapter Four, I described ways of improving your benefit/cost ratio by increasing the benefits. In this chapter, I will suggest ways to improve it by reducing the costs. Note that I said, "reducing," not "eliminating," the costs. Fitness activities—like many other worthwhile activities—are not cost-free. Still, you can make them less costly. Given the abundant benefits of a fitness lifestyle over its alternatives, a cost reduction may be all you need to tip the balance in favor of the benefits and keep you motivated. My goals in this chapter are to alert you to some costs and help you reduce them.

SOLUTIONS

Money matters.

The first and most obvious category is "financial costs." These costs include items you buy, such as running shoes or a bicycle, gym membership fees, and instructional costs like for a personal trainer or a class. Costs can range from as low as a hundred dollars up to several thousand dollars. How much will be determined partly by your choice of fitness activity. Walking, starting from your front door, probably only requires a pair of good shoes. Lifting weights and running on a treadmill in an inexpensive gym can be low cost. However, safety in a gym requires familiarity with equipment and techniques. If problems lead to injuries, the bargain may be a poor one, so balance in the possible financial costs with the possible aggravation of injury when considering how much to "indulge" or "economize" on your choice of a gym, a personal trainer or even a pair of running shoes. The most expensive isn't always going to be the most risk-free, nor is the least expensive alternative always going to be the most risky. Check relevant certifications, solicit references from people you trust, and shop around.

Also, once properly instructed, consider economical home alternatives. For example, after thinking through our needs, Carolyn and I made a fitness room out of what used to be our house's basement coal room. The total cost for paint, free weights, playroom-type rubber floor pads, and a few pieces of miscellaneous apparatus (some of which we made) totaled less than $400. Over the twenty years we've been using it, we've continued to add or replace equipment, but the room has saved us a lot in both money and time, considering the fees and travel time that a fitness center would have required.

Managing time costs.

Time costs will be your second major commitment. Scheduling in everything you consider important within the 24-hour day can be difficult, if not impossible. If your fitness program crowds out another activity that's important to you, you are experiencing a time cost, and you may need to reassess your priorities.

While fitness activities should be an important part of your life, other areas deserve your time and attention too. If your spiritual life, your intellectual pursuits, families and relationships, career, and other personal interests that give your life meaning and purpose are slighted, you will eventually feel out of balance. On the other hand, if all of these important areas are attended to at some reasonable level, you should function well. Thus, one theme implicit throughout this chapter is to honor all important areas of your life—in a reasonable balance.[10] If your fitness activity causes an imbalance in some other area, the cost will eventually feel too high and your motivation will suffer.

Think of time as a finite resource. In allocating it, first assign high priorities to adequate rest and nutrition. Think of your body and your mind as analogous to a water fountain. If there is no water going into a fountain, there can be no water coming out of it. Like the fountain that gives water to thirsty people, imagine nutrient intake and your rest as energy available for the important areas of your life. If you aren't getting enough rest and nutrients—and getting them consistently—you will become like a fountain without enough water coming in. Eventually fatigue will increase the discomfort of your mental and physical activities and numb the benefits you get from your efforts. So avoid letting a fitness activity or any other activity routinely infringe on your rest, and avoid letting a weight reduction goal unduly restrict your nutrient intake.

For long-term success, figure out what activities are important to you and then give higher priority to them than to less important alternatives. Good time managers don't always do more things than poor time managers, but they make certain that they do more of the things they consider important. As a result, they feel more satisfaction. If an activity seems less important, good time managers give it lower priority and less time: They simply don't do it, they do it in a minimally adequate way, or they have someone else do it.

Ask yourself two questions when trying to decide whether an activity deserves higher or lower priority:

First, is this task important, or is it merely urgent?[11] An important activity is one you believe is really worth doing. In contrast, an urgent activity is one that you feel pressured to do soon. If the urgent activity is also important, it probably deserves very high priority. However, if it is not, it probably deserves low priority, despite the pressure you feel to do it. Filing income tax returns before the deadline is both urgent and important and deserves high priority. You might want to skip your morning swim on tax day to meet the deadline. Going to your neighbor's garage sale before the bargains get snapped up by someone else may feel urgent, but may not be very important; in this case, your morning swim probably deserves the higher priority

Second, is this task important to you, or is it just important to someone else who shouldn't be having that much influence on you anyway? For example, imagine a man choosing between taking daily walks and keeping his house spotlessly clean. If the only concern for the spotless house is the criticism of an over-bearing relative, the man—if he is a good time manager—will make sure his daily walk always happens and may do only a minimal job on his housecleaning much of the time.

You may find it helpful to write down the tasks and activities that compete for your time. Seeing them on paper can decrease the chances of overlooking anything. Such a list can make it easier for you to prioritize each item on its relative importance vs urgency and on its relevance to you vs someone else.

When you give activities attention according to their importance, you will get more done on things that you truly care about. Beyond that, acting on clear priorities can reduce the costs of fitness in either of two ways. On one hand, if you decide that the fitness activity is more important, and you reduce the time you spend on the competing activity, you have less feeling of loss because you've thought your priorities through. If you decide that the competing activity is more important, and reduce your time on the fitness activity, you again have less loss. In this latter case, however, I'd still encourage you to do *some* fitness activity, in line with the idea that some activity is better than none at all. Many benefits can still happen, albeit at a slower rate. Whichever activity gets more of your time, the cost/benefit ratio for the fitness activity can be more favorable than if you didn't think through your priorities.

Conflicts between fitness and some important areas of life can be more apparent than real. After re-examining the conflict, you may realize that you don't need to choose one over the other. Jim's experience provides a good example of this: During his undergraduate years, Jim studied hard. He also took time each day for exercise and he enjoyed feeling fit. However, when he began graduate school, he was overwhelmed by all the homework his professors assigned, and he decided that he didn't have time to both take workouts and study. He was just too busy.

Unfortunately, things didn't improve. He studied hard, but he wasn't getting enough done and he was disappointed with his test scores. At the end of his first semester, he still had two papers to complete before starting the second semester, so he continued to work on those during the semester break.

Happily, Jim also decided to "indulge" himself during the break by taking a workout each day. It felt like an "indulgence" because, after all, the total time for a workout—considering going to and from the gym, changing clothes before and after the workout, doing the workout itself and the shower—took two hours out of each day.

To his surprise, however, Jim found that by taking this two-hour "indulgence" he actually made gains in his productivity. That is, for the rest of any day that included a workout, he was able to read more, remember it better, and be more creative in how he integrated material for his papers. He got more done because of his two-hour "indulgences" and he felt better too. Instead of thinking that he didn't have time to take workouts, he now concluded that he didn't have time to omit workouts. The rest of his graduate career was more productive and also more pleasant.

Exercise gave Jim the more popular benefits of fitness, but he got added value in terms of the way the rest of each day went too. He became more efficient and more effective as a scholar. Other people who previously felt they were "too busy" have found other value-added benefits from exercise: more patience for the supervisor of a slightly rebellious, albeit bright and productive staff; more consistency and calm for the mother of two pre-school children; more mental flexibility and energy for the computer programmer; and so on. Like Jim, many people have learned that they don't have time to omit exercise. Once you try it you may find that you don't either.

Attending to your comforts is important. You shouldn't give them all up just because you want to get fit. For example, several times I've referred to people taking early morning walks or early morning swims. Early morning exercise means only showering and dressing for the day once, which can reduce a time cost. Still, there's nothing sacred about what time you choose to exercise. Maybe you aren't a morning person. If that's the case, choose another time of day, and enjoy a different reduction in cost. Similarly, if you have a favorite TV show at a certain time or like to have coffee with a friend at a certain time, choose a different time to exercise.

The fewer comforts you give up, the fewer costs you pay for exercise. There is nothing virtuous about needless deprivation. Stack the cards in favor of fitness by honoring as many of your usual comforts as possible. Initially writing out a schedule is quite likely to help you consider all your options.

Reducing physical costs.
Physical discomforts can—and often do—initially result from a fitness activity. Perhaps the most obvious ones would be fatigue and pains in your muscles, joints or ligaments that can occur during or after exercise. These should be temporary as your body adjusts to a new regime, but they are real.

My main concern here is pacing—regulating your level of difficulty or challenge. In Chapter Four, I suggested that you set your fitness activities at optimal levels of difficulty, so that your efforts feel both satisfying and worthwhile. If you instead set the level too low or too high, you may suffer from boredom or from feeling overwhelmed. Unfortunately, you could have worse consequences: Most notably, if you set the difficulty level too high and then try to follow through, you may end up very sore or very tired, or with injuries requiring a break for a period of recovery. Such costs can be devastating to your motivation. Despite what your weekend warrior friends may say about "no pain, no gain," I'd instead endorse the wisdom of *The Tortoise and The Hare* fable: "Slow and steady wins the race." Set up a mildly challenging routine that you can continue, and increase the demand only after your body is ready to continue at a higher level.

I hope you share my enthusiasm for the idea of people maximizing their potentials. The trouble is that we rarely know what our potentials are, and denial can be a hindrance in getting an accurate estimate. We need to pay attention to our legitimate physical limitations.

Are you older than you used to be? A dumb question, but it might be relevant if you are in denial. Do you have a disability? Maybe a bad knee? Maybe too much weight? A heart condition? None of these things are crimes, and depending on the exercises you choose, they may not be much of a hindrance as you work your way to better fitness. On the other hand, if you choose wrongly, ignoring some relevant physical limitation, you are going to pay a high cost and perhaps quit.

Alan learned this the hard way. Alan ran middle-distance track in high school and college, and ran in 5K road races in his thirties and forties. Then he injured his right hip in an accident and had to have a hip replacement. Alan's doctor predicted that he would have problems if he tried to run with his new hip, and encouraged him to instead bike or swim for exercise. Unfortunately, Alan ignored that advice, resumed running and injured himself again. After another operation and some physical rehabilitation, he came to terms with his physical limitation and took up biking. He remains fit today.

Alan suffered a lot of needless frustration and pain before he acknowledged his limitation and took up biking. It isn't his preferred exercise, but it is better for him now than running had become, and far, far better than doing nothing. Of course, many opt for doing nothing under such circumstances. If you're in an analogous situation, look at alternatives with an open mind. What you end up with may not be what you initially preferred, but you can gear your expectations to the new benefits while enjoying the lowered costs in the meantime. You're not that old! (I address physical limitation issues in more detail in Chapter Nine.)

Reducing Psychological Costs.
The most obvious psychological discomforts/costs that can accompany fitness activities are boredom, frustration, and competition-derived ego-threat.

I've touched on boredom a bit already, suggesting that you set the difficulty of your exercise at an optimally challenging level, rather than making it too easy. Concerning other remedies, many people eliminate boredom by switching to a different type of activity. For example, if swimming bores you, consider biking. Other people find it helpful to vary their concurrent stimulation, whether by working out with friends, working out with music, altering the environment where they exercise (e.g., following new walking routes), or adding some skill goals (see Chapter Four). My remaining suggestion regarding boredom would be to reschedule your exercise to a time of day when it can be a welcome contrast to some predictable stress or chaos that you experience at work or at home. Properly placed, a workout that otherwise might seem boring can feel like a welcome immersion into a stress-free place and time. Since no one will call you or ask you to take on one more task during your workout, it can provide a refuge or a decompression time.

Concerning frustration, I should first point out that mild frustration can be somewhat motivating. It can be the uncomfortable feeling that you are willing to work hard enough to get rid of by performing better. Too often, however, frustration is simply another cost that makes you want to quit.

A more constructive approach to frustration comes from addressing its main cause—unrealistic expectations. People become frustrated when something they try to accomplish doesn't happen the way they (unrealistically) expected it to.

Jill had this problem: Jill began a weight-loss program that involved both diet and exercise, and lost several pounds each week during the first month. Naturally, she expected to keep on losing at that rate. Several months later, when she had to face the fact that she wasn't losing weight as rapidly as before, she felt frustrated and discouraged. The problem wasn't her adherence to her program; rather, it was her expectations. She expected something that simply doesn't happen very often. A weight loss expert could have told her that the pounds almost always come off more quickly at first, and much more slowly later on. A consultation with a personal trainer clarified this for Jill, after which she regained her motivation and proceeded with her program.

Whether you are trying to improve your general fitness, lose weight or increase your strength, you can minimize your frustration by gearing your expectations to be in tune with realistic pacing, realistic patterns of progress and realistic goals.

Concerning ego-derived competition threat,[12] it is important to realize that you've been in competitive situations all your life, situations where your performance on something was compared with someone else's. For example, did you learn to talk sooner than Cousin Harriet? Which one of you learned to ride a bicycle first? Which of you was the better student? Which of you was more popular in high school? Which of you has the higher status job? Which of you has the better adjusted child? And, of course, which of you is more fit?

Competitions can have either good or bad effects on people. Let's begin with the bad effects. Suppose Jerry has just won the city tennis tournament, and most people there agree he's a better player than any of his fellow competitors. If, because of being a better tennis player, Jerry now seems to be judged by some people to be a better person, and if he takes such judgments seriously, his ego is more likely to feel threatened next time he competes—after all, no one can win all the time and no one wants to feel like a less good person. Of course, a similar feeling of threat can be predicted for any of the players—not just Jerry—who takes such judgments seriously. Under repeated judgments like this—and in our society, there are many repeats—Jerry and his fellow competitors can develop what is called an "ego-orientation" toward competition, an orientation that focuses more on protecting the ego against threat and less on the enjoyment of the game or the enjoyment of figuring out how to improve it. I wouldn't recommend ego-oriented competition if you are interested in building a stable sense of self worth—and in the meantime, it's not much fun.

Now, imagine a different scenario where Jerry and his fellow players think that winning and losing have nothing to do with which players are better or worse as people—only as players. Here, each person still wants to win, but the stakes are less overwhelming. Their egos aren't threatened. With less concern for their egos, the competition and the efforts leading up to that competition can be constructive and fun, win or lose.

Here's why: When we are free of threats and other discomforts, urges within us push for mastery of various "tasks" we choose—tasks involving athletics, our jobs, relationships or other matters. We naturally feel satisfaction as we make progress toward task mastery. Practices can be fun. Also, we feel satisfaction when we see new indications of that mastery during competitions, whether we win or lose—so competitions can be fun too.

When you are at your most ego-oriented extreme, it may be difficult to comprehend athletes who say they enjoy workouts, or scholars who say they enjoy studying, or business people who say they enjoy going to work. You might be even more skeptical hearing such people say they look forward to the next tournament, the next exam, or the next job interview—occasions which can provide chances to see how they've progressed and see ways they can improve even more.

The urge for task mastery (and the satisfaction you can get from pursuing it) is natural. You don't have to learn it. Unfortunately, if you are too immersed in an ego orientation, you can get out of touch with this urge. The good news is that with patience you can get it back.

In contrast to the term "ego orientation," research-ers call the approach toward competition that focuses on developing skills the "task orientation" to competition. People with task orientations enjoy many advantages over people with ego orientations. Those advantages include the following:

First, task oriented people find competition and other challenges less threatening. As a result, they are free enough of fear to engage in tasks and to *persist* at them until they become proficient, rather than quit.

Second, task oriented people are open to more ways to improve. Here's why: as with other anxieties, people under ego threat develop tunnel vision and hesitate to try new approaches. They may not be happy with their current results, but what if they did even more poorly by trying something new? Wouldn't that be terrible? Not terrible for task oriented people; they would simply consider it as "data" to learn from. Task oriented people are more free to risk experimenting with approaches that could fail.

Third, task oriented people can look at the accomplishments of others and be encouraged, rather than discouraged. They can say, "If that person can do it, maybe some day I can too!" In fact, they can look at competitors as allies rather than as adversaries—"Their successes can spur me on, and I can help them too."

Fourth, task oriented people are not discouraged when they aren't instantly successful. For the ego-oriented person, anything but instant success can be a threat; after all, it's a threat if others are "better," even if only temporarily. Consequently, the ego-oriented competitor places much value on having an innate ability for the task; if they don't think they are unusually blessed, they are more likely to quit—"I'm just not cut out for this." Of course, task-oriented competitors prefer to have innate ability too, but their big emphasis is on being able to persist and improve—only with persistence can people most fully develop their potentials, whether those potentials are high or low. And development is what it's all about for the task oriented person.

Fifth, task oriented people get more enjoyment and satisfaction from their activities. This is true partly because they are more likely to stay with their activities long enough to enjoy the fruits of their labor. But there is an additional reason: Contrary to what TV ads would have you believe, meaningful satisfaction doesn't come from commodities (stuff) you buy and then passively consume. Think about it: Do you get meaningful satisfaction by passively consuming chemicals, watching sit-coms, buying new cars, or being in relationships where only the other person is trying to make it work? You might get temporary enjoyment, but not much more.

More likely, when you get meaningful satisfaction, you get it indirectly—as a by-product of endeavors you believe to be worth doing and which you are actively involved in.[13] But it is hard to be actively involved—and to stay actively involved rather than quit—if you always feel that your ego is on the line. That's not a problem when you adopt a task orientation to the activity.

Again, competition *per se* is neither good nor bad. Judging your worth as a person on the basis of your performance can lead you to an ego orientation and a number of bad consequences. Keeping your evaluations of yourself independent of your performances can enable you to adopt a task orientation and a number of more fortunate consequences. Given the nature of our society, you may not have had much choice about which orientation to adopt as you grew up. I hope you'll find ways to exert your independent choice from here on and choose in favor of a task orientation.

To help you follow through with that choice, begin by telling yourself three main things:

(1) Each time you find yourself thinking or behaving in an ego-oriented way, remind yourself that your worth as a person is a positive, unearned "given" which is equal to that of any other person. Even if "Tom" is a highly effective politician, or if "Dick" is the most attractive man on the planet, or if "Harry" is the richest, your worth as a human remains equal to theirs, whether they think so or not. Similarly, if your Cousin Harriet is more fit than you, your worth as a human remains equal to hers, whether her mother thinks so or not.

(2) Also remind yourself that that your worth is unchangeable. It stays the same regardless of your next achievements, attributes, wealth, situation

or lack thereof. It is not on the line no matter how often you fail and have to start over.

(3) Don't expect to change from your ego orientation quickly. This mental habit was shaped by many forces over a long period of time. Just keep reminding yourself and be patient.

Reducing social costs.

When I addressed "time costs," I emphasized the importance of balancing all of your needs. One of those needs is for social interaction. If your fitness program takes up time and energy that you really want to spend on your social life, your motivation for fitness will eventually suffer.

Beyond what I've already said about this, the main suggestion I want to add is to consult with your significant others about any changes in routine which might inconvenience or otherwise affect them. Avoid surprising them and they'll probably become your allies. Probably. (In Chapter Ten, I go into detail on how to deal with people who, instead of being allies, place unanticipated costs or even obstacles in the way of your fitness program.)

Springboard.

The following questions address some of the cost concerns in this chapter. I suggest you write out and date your answers so that you can re-evaluate them as you progress.

1. Are your choices regarding your type of exercise and related expenses in keeping with your financial resources and priorities?
    Yes ___ No ___
2. Is your fitness program in balance with the other important areas of your life?
    Yes ___ No ___
3. With your fitness program, are you able to maintain adequate amounts of bed rest and nutrient intake, and on a consistent schedule?
    Yes ___ No ___
4. With the fitness program you've developed, are there some "fun" or "comforting" activities still included?
    Yes ___ No ___
5. When you make increases in your exercise level, do you make them gradually?
    Yes ___ No ___
6. Is your exercise program in keeping with your physical limitations?
    Yes ___ No ___
7. Are your exercise sessions adequately free of boredom and frustration?
    Yes ___ No ___
8. Are your exercise sessions adequately free of ego threat?
    Yes ___ No ___

9. Is your fitness program adequately free of social loss or aggravation?

    Yes ___ No ___

For any question where your answer is "No," I hope you'll reread the pertinent section of this chapter, think about ways you might improve your situation, and write down specific steps to make that happen. Then try implementing those steps. Regardless of the outcome, return later to what you've written, consider modifications, and repeat the process.

C H A P T E R   6

STRENGTHENING YOUR PLANS

The Problem: Target Time Drifts: Critical lapses in your motivation and follow- through.

THE LONG-TERM SUCCESS of your fitness program depends on: (1) its benefits outweighing its costs, (2) your expectations of success and (3) your having plans and structures that are relatively easy to follow through on. In everyday life, unexpected elements can converge to temporarily distort your perception of the relevant costs, benefits, and expectations, or make your plans or structures hard to follow.

When this happens, you may suffer temporary lapses in your program. Crucial adjustments may be in order. You may need to alter the plans and structures that make your fitness activity happen almost automatically, without requiring daily conflicts and decisions.

This chapter addresses the troublesome lapses that I call "Target Time Drifts," and the adjustments you can make to get past them. With Target Time Drifts, you may feel motivated to stay with the fitness plan most of the time, maybe even 23 out of each day's 24 hours. Then, unfortunately, you lose that motivation at the most relevant time, at Target Time, that time when you meant to take your walk, go for a run, or whatever other activity. These lapses are not character flaws. Chastising yourself won't help. Working out a new approach that gets you safely past debilitating decision points will.

Let's consider Donald's case. Donald set up a program that would establish a fitness lifestyle for himself. He decided to take up swimming on a regular basis. It was in the fall, he had just moved to a new job in a new town, and his apartment was a short, four-block walk from a nice indoor pool. The pool opened for lap swimming at 6 a.m. each day, giving Donald an opportunity to exercise early, before interruptions, and still have time for everything else in his new, busy life.

Donald's early morning swims went well for the first month. Unfortunately, they took a belly flop with the season's first significant cold spell. On that first chilly morning, Donald awoke and realized that he would be much more comfortable staying in bed. As he lay there images flashed through his mind of the cold floor meeting his bare feet and of the cold room as he stood in his pajamas, deciding what to wear. Then he thought about finding his swimming gear and finding his keys, a warm jacket and gloves. He could almost feel the cold wind hitting him as he imagined walking to the pool, and the chill of first getting into the water. That chill was always the worst part of the whole workout, and now he imagined how he'd be doing it with a lowered core body temperature because of the cold walk. In his semi-awake state, he asked himself if he really wanted to swim or to just sack in for another hour, and guess what? He chose the latter.

The extra sleep felt OK, but in truth Donald wasn't very happy with himself when he finally got up, just in time to go to work. Several times during the day he berated himself for having "wimped out," and he stayed in a less-than-cheerful mood all day long. Not surprisingly, he made a resolution to swim the next morning, no matter what kind of weather.

But he made that resolution when he was awake and warm. When next morning came, Donald had a repeat of the previous day's images and again went back to sleep, foregoing his swim. He also repeated the self-chastisement and resolution-making later in the day—but to no avail. After several more days of not making it to the pool, he decided that maybe he wasn't a cold-weather swimmer and that perhaps he'd take it up again in the spring, when the weather got better. Meanwhile, he rationalized, his new job was giving him plenty to do.

Donald's problem started as an example of Target Time Drift. He went through most of each day motivated to swim the next morning. For most hours of those days, he realized that the benefits outweighed the costs. He knew his previous swims had given him ample reason to expect future success. The only time he wasn't motivated was when his alarm went off. Then the costs (the cold floor, the initial chill of the water, and so on) loomed large in Donald's mind. The memories of how good he felt during and after his swims seemed very remote. After several days of failure, his expectations of success in even getting out of bed on time went down, but his self-chastisements continued to be painful. Gradually, his motivational problem became more than just Target Time Drift. That is, he lost his inclination to even think about swimming, at least for the rest of the winter.

Target Time Drift is something everyone is vulnerable to, although, of course, the Drift doesn't always involve the weather or early morning swims. For example,

- Luke's friends pressure him to skip his runs and join them for beers after work.
- Julia feels pulled to TV sit-coms when she would normally lift weights.
- Larry feels the urge to skip his noonday walks when writing big reports.

Target Time Drift is normal, but it doesn't have to undermine your overall motivation and progress. Once in a while, it may actually be more appropriate to skip the exercise and stay in bed, have a beer with friends, see a TV show, or work through the noon-hour. Perhaps the cost/benefit ratios of one's life may temporarily change in such ways that it would be needlessly rigid to stick to the exercise plans on that day. The problem comes when Target Time Drift happens too often, and when the overall cost/benefit ratios in fact would favor doing the fitness activity.

SOLUTIONS

When you wish you could resist the Target Time Drift and stay with your fitness plan you need something better than self-chastisement and new resolutions. Neither the self-chastisements nor the resolutions—by themselves—provide the implementation steps you need to get your workout going. "Just do it!" can be a helpful slogan once you are envisioning the favorable cost/benefit ratios at Target Time and envisioning a sequence of useful, possible steps to "just do." But before that, "Just do it!" is merely hot air that can leave you groping without direction and feeling bad. Instead, consider the following approaches:

Look for Patterns.
What happened differently when you had Target Time Drift that didn't happen on days when you succeeded in following your plan? Is there a pattern? The pattern, if there is one, may help you more directly pinpoint factors you can change. Using the above examples,

Luke may be more vulnerable to pressures from friends on days when his running partner can't join him anyway.

Julia may find the TV more tempting only on days she's expecting a call from her romantic partner.

Larry's urge to work over the noon-hour might be stronger if he hasn't reached a good stopping spot in the report he's writing.

Some good solutions are amazingly obvious once you've identified the pattern. It may be fairly easy for Luke to get a more consistent running partner, or for Julia to make clear phone arrangements with her romantic partner, or for Larry to watch for a stopping spot from 11:30 on. If he reaches one before 12:00, maybe he can reward himself by taking off early.

Of course, adjustments may be more complicated. For example, Larry's boss may have problems with him taking off early, in which case he may reward himself instead with light, easily interruptible tasks until noon. Alternatively, if, before noon, the section of the report he's on is one that has no good stopping spot for at least another hour, maybe he can spend the last ten minutes of the morning jotting down an outline of what he'll write after his walk—and then leave. It's a safe bet that Larry will return ready to do better work than if he'd toiled on with no refreshing break.

Apply a Benefit Reminder.
If relatively easy solutions like these don't get you past Target Time Drift, try going back to basics: Look again at

the reasons you decided to establish a fitness lifestyle in the first place. Perhaps those reasons are getting undermined during your Target Time Drift. The patterns and challenges you noticed may give you clues as to how that happened.

Something may have happened that made the benefits seem relatively remote or unimportant while at the same time making the costs seem to multiply. Compare the perceptions you have of the cost/benefit ratios during the rest of the day, when your motivation is back, to your perception of those ratios during the Drift time. Keep in mind that your goals are for your life, not for one day. Then ask yourself, "Which is the distorted perception?" If the perception you have during the motivated 23 hours of the day is the distorted one (for example, suppose you actually hate your chosen exercise, but are in denial about that during most of the day), you'll do well to change your fitness program (for example, by choosing a more agreeable exercise).

On the other hand, if the distortion is with the Target Time perception, write yourself a Benefit Reminder. A Benefit Reminder is a brief, truthful statement that reminds you of the reasons you are doing fitness activities in the first place. Read and say this Benefit Reminder to yourself whenever you need to place the valid perception foremost your mind. Continuing with the above examples,

Donald could have said to himself, "This cold air feels lousy now, but I'll feel fine once I've swum half a lap, and I'll feel even better for the rest of the day!"

Luke, whose friends want him to join them for a beer instead of run might say, "I want my stomach smaller, not larger!"

Julia, wrestling between the TV show and weight lifting might say, "I'll have more energy for fun if I work out instead of sitting around waiting for that call."

As for choosing between more office work and a noon-hour walk, Larry might say, "Walking helps keep me from burn-out and increases my afternoon's productivity."

Mentally repeat your Benefit Reminder any time you waver. ANY time! It will help you see through the temporary distortions and remember the important benefits.

Set up an automatic Drift Override.[14]
Your brain is an incredible marvel, but during Target Time Drifts, it can work against your best interests, providing you with seemingly legitimate justifications for going off-target and missing your exercise. For such times, I recommend an automatic procedure that overrides these self-directed con-jobs. This procedure involves four concepts: Target Time Intentions, Decision Points, Target-Relevant Actions, and Prompts.

A Target Time Intention is your goal to be "on target" at target time. For Donald, a target time intention could be "to arrive at the swimming pool at 6 a.m." The justification and strength behind a target-time intention comes from its relevance to larger, more important goals, such as "to feel better for the rest of the day," or "to get fit." The target-time intention won't be strong without strong commitment to these higher- level goals.

Decision Points are situations along your path to the target, troublesome forks in the road, so to speak, where you are most vulnerable to taking a wrong turn. Knowing the pattern of your Target Time Drift can help you identify these Decision Points or forks. In Donald's case, the most troublesome situation came as soon as the alarm went off—instead of automatically getting out of bed, he listened to his sleep-fogged brain and chose to linger under the covers, rationalize about the cold, and then to go back to sleep.

Target-Relevant Actions are actions you take at Decision Points that keep you moving toward the target. For Donald, when the alarm went off, Target Relevant Actions would have included putting his feet on the floor, standing up, going to where his clothes are kept, and getting dressed. Doing these things fairly quickly would have gotten him past the tempting alternative of staying in bed.

Prompts are brief, pre-rehearsed summaries of the Actions you want to take at the Decision Points. Prompts take the form of, "When X happens, I do Y!" where X is the Decision Point and Y is the Target-Relevant Action. For Donald, the Prompt could have been, "When the alarm goes off, I get out of bed and get dressed!" Saying the Prompt at the Decision Point helps initiate and strengthen the Target-Relevant Action; saying it also helps you avoid getting sidetracked with non-relevant actions. Most notably, Prompts help you move quickly past the Decision Points, acting somewhat automatically on the decisions you made earlier, when your thinking and perception were less distorted.

Using these four concepts to set up an effective Drift Override requires advance preparation. A crucial start comes with your recognition of your Drift problem and your identification of its pattern. From there, you can work out how each of these concepts applies to you. Write down your Target Time Intention, your Decision Point(s), and your corresponding Target-Relevant Action(s). Then compose and write down your Prompt(s). Before your next attempt to overcome the Drift, review what you've written and rehearse the Prompt(s). Don't expect these concepts and their applications to "naturally" be at your fingertips when in the next vulnerable situation—not yet, anyway. So again, rehearse well before you reach Target Time.

Beyond getting yourself ready to apply the four concepts, knowing your pattern can help you identify and eliminate other problems ahead of time. For example, suppose Donald realizes that he bogs down and gets distracted when choosing what he'll wear to the pool or looking for his keys or packing his swim bag. Taking care of these things the night before, when his head is clear, would make for fewer Decision Points during his early morning fog. The fewer, the better, since each time he has to choose or decide opens the possibility of going off target.

Also, don't be surprised if other derailing situations pop up over time. For example, suppose that after Donald again gets consistent at getting up, getting dressed and out of the house on time, his boss develops a penchant for sending out late night emails. Suppose further that with his boss's change, Donald's urge to check the inbox before swimming has become nearly irresistible. Worse still, giving in has led to checking other messages as well as those from the boss, to having a cup of coffee while contemplating his responses, and ultimately to using up the time that had been dedicated to swimming. As with his previous Drift, Donald regrets this later on each day, realizing that the emails could have waited until after his swim. Having the same Target Time Intention as before, he can regroup, composing a new Prompt like, "When I go past my computer (Decision Point), I ignore it and leave the house (Target-Relevant Action)." The Drift Override approach can work for a lot of situations where your program is vulnerable.

A note on structures and freedom.
You are not alone if by now you find yourself objecting to solutions involving Patterns, Benefit Reminders and Drift Overrides. You may consider their application too rigidly lockstep—an affront to your freedom.

If so, I encourage you to think of freedom in terms of (1) informed choices (choices based on adequate information) and (2) the ability to follow through on those choices. Your freedom is greatest when you are able to make and follow through on informed choices regarding matters important to you. When your intentions get hi-jacked by last minute distractions and impulses, you aren't free. You're getting jerked about like someone else's puppet. For Donald, it was more important to swim than to stay in bed, but he didn't have the freedom to clearly choose or act on that preference. His distorted, unbalanced perspective during the Target Time Drifts robbed him of it. If, by applying the above "lockstep" structures, he got himself to the pool on time, these structures—despite all their regimentation—would have increased his freedom. If your choices and your follow-through get enhanced by the concepts of this chapter, they will have increased your freedom too.

Springboard.
The following questions and actions will help you control your Target Time Drift. Your responses will have more

chance of helping you if you write them down, think about them, and revise them as you attack the Drift.

1. Patterns:
    a. What sequence of steps does your Target Time Drift seem to follow?
    b. Can any of these steps be altered to provide a quick, easy solution?
2. Benefit Reminders:
    a. What are your reasons for wanting a fitness lifestyle? What do you hope it will give you?
    b. From these reasons, write out a brief Benefit Reminder. Make and rehearse a plan to say this Reminder to yourself any time you feel likely to "drift."
3. Drift Overrides:
    a. Justified by your reasons (benefits), compose a Target Time Intention that has the goal of getting past your Drift and into your program each day by a specific time. Write it down to increase your ease of recall.
    b. Identify your Decision Points, situations where you are most vulnerable to getting "off-target." (When possible, reduce the number of Decision Points—i.e., places where you might be vulnerable to going off-track. Using Donald's case for an example, he could reduce

his Decision Points by packing his swim bag and selecting his clothes the night before.)

c. Identify Target-Relevant Actions to take at these Decision Points.

d. Compose a Prompt that summarizes what Target-Relevant Action to take at each Decision Point—"When X happens, I do Y!"

e. Rehearse, and then use the Prompt(s). That is, when you arrive at each Decision Point, say the corresponding Prompt to support you as you follow through on your pre-determined choice of action—and keep on target! Let it become your automatic response.

PART III
INCREASING YOUR READINESS
TO RESPOND TO LIFE'S CHALLENGES

C H A P T E R   7

BOUNCE

Effective Recovery From Interruptions

The Problem: Extended Interruptions can foil motivation.
NO ONE'S FITNESS program is immune to extended interruptions. Sooner or later, no matter how well you plan
your life, you'll have an injury, an illness, a vacation, a
surge in job demands or some other circumstance that
will interfere. The problem is that even if the interruption lasts only a couple of weeks, it can lead to your program's collapse.

So if it is impossible to devise an interruption-free
program, what can you do to keep fit regardless of interruptions? The answer is Bounce. Bounce is the process
of effectively coming back from an interruption. In the
long term, the quality of your fitness program isn't going
to depend as much on how perfectly you follow your daily
plan—i.e., no extended interruptions—as on how well
you bounce back into the routine once the interruption
is over.

Clarissa's story illustrates several of the problems
of a significant interruption and its aftermath. Clarissa

83

had been a steady swimmer for over a year. Five mornings each week she was in the pool at six o'clock sharp regardless of rain, sunshine, ice or snow. She swam when she was busy and she swam even when she was tired. She always felt better after her swim. Some days she swam a mile freestyle; other days, she did sprints; other days she did various strokes at various speeds and distances. She was a good swimmer and enjoyed getting better.

Then something happened that was totally beyond her control: The Aquatic Center's "pool pack" broke down. The pool pack was the pool's "brains," the computerized water quality control system for the pool, regulating both the water's temperature and its chemical composition. It took the Aquatic Center seven months to diagnose the problem, order a new custom pool pack, receive it, install it, and test it. During that time the pool was closed and Clarissa did not swim.

Neither did she do any other exercise. She kept thinking that the pool pack problem wouldn't last very long, and that this was a good chance to catch up on other things—her garden, her sewing closet, her photo album, the garage sale she'd been putting off. She also didn't mind occasionally going to bed later and sleeping later the next morning. She liked swimming, but these other things were nice too.

Finally, the pool was up and operating again. Clarissa didn't go back on the opening day because this "swim time" would give her just enough time before work to finish a sewing project she had started. She did swim the second day, but to do it she had to cancel a breakfast meeting with several friends, which wasn't pleasant. To make things worse, her swim was unexpectedly difficult: she felt out of rhythm and she was slow. Halfway through what would have been a typical mile seven months earlier, she was exhausted and ready to quit. She was tired for the rest of the day. On the third morning it was very hard for her to drag herself to the pool to do it all over again. The thought of trying a mile again was pretty distasteful, so she decided to try sprints. They went badly too, and later on that day she found herself with a sore shoulder. On the fourth morning, she got up in time to swim, thought about it for a minute and went back to bed. On the fifth day, she got up in time, but instead did housework in preparation for her mother-in-law's visit later in the day.

Her mother-in-law's visit gave her some welcome time off from the thought of swimming. When the visit was over Clarissa gave the pool another try. Unfortunately, she further aggravated her shoulder problem. Over the next few weeks, many swims got cancelled for other priorities, and the days she did swim were marked with increased shoulder pain and excessive fatigue. Finally, when it was time to renew her pool pass for another month, Clarissa asked herself, "Is this really worth it?"— and answered, "No."

At various times over the next year, Clarissa regretted her decision. On the other hand, the longer she stayed away, the harder it was to picture herself in a lifestyle that could accommodate swimming. Also, she had doubts about whether her body still could take steady exercise, regardless of whether her schedule could.

SOLUTIONS

Several things converged to work against Clarissa's swimming routine and ultimately against her motivation to stay with it. The trigger for her problems was the interruption—the time away from swimming while the pool was closed for repair. However, her alternative activities during the interruption and the way she resumed her program were the real problems.

Having a Plan B.
For most people an extended interruption doesn't simply mean a drop-off in the preferred exercise. It also means a change in the basic routine. A vacuum is created—and vacuums can lead to new lifestyles.

In Clarissa's case, for example, when she stopped swimming, she did other things in the mornings when she chose to, and often she stayed up later, knowing she'd have more time to sleep next morning. These other activities were enjoyable, and by the time the pool was operating again, she had lost fitness, making these other activities even more compelling choices. After all, they were certainly preferable to the soreness and excessive fatigue that swimming gave her now. My first guideline addresses the sort of "vacuum problem" Clarissa faced: Have a Plan B for when you can't follow Plan A.

For Clarissa, Plan A was swimming. When the pool wasn't operating, whether for a day, a week, or seven months, Plan B could have been walking, biking, rollerblading, running, joining a Zumba class or an early morning step aerobics class. Any of these exercises could have served two important functions. The first, of course, would be that of keeping Clarissa fit and less vulnerable to fatigue and injury once she got back to swimming. The second function—especially if she did the Plan B exercise during her previous swim time—would be that of a "placeholder." This Plan B/placeholder would make that time more easily convert back to "swim time." Swimming wouldn't have to compete with new habits (such as sleeping-in instead of going to bed earlier), social expectations (such as breakfasts with friends instead of coffee with them later), and routines (such as housework early instead of housework at other times of day). Unfortunately, by the time the pool was ready again, Clarissa instead had to make more changes than just resuming swimming, and that was hard.

Reassessing after interruptions.
My second guideline for an effective bounce is to do a self-assessment after the interruption ends. In terms of fitness, Clarissa was not the same person after the

seven-month layoff that she was before. Similarly, she would not have been the same person after a nasty bout of bronchitis or a two-week Caribbean cruise. Since she was, in effect, a different person, she needed to begin her return to swimming with a fresh self-assessment and a new workout plan based on that assessment.

To start with, she should have set the difficulty level of her first swim much lower than her previous level and paid close attention to the impact of that effort over the next several days. Next, if she found herself unduly tired or sore, she should have allowed herself to recuperate and then experiment with even lower difficulty levels, repeating the recuperations and lowerings until she found a comfortable starting point. From there she could set up a plan of gradual increases in difficulty, never over-reaching her readiness to advance.

Instead, Clarissa tried to resume swimming at her old level of intensity, and with a fraction of her previous fitness. No wonder her body rebelled! She needed weeks to return more gently to her previous stamina and strength. Perhaps she also needed to rebuild mental tolerance for the more strenuous activity. Thus, my second guideline for an effective bounce is to do a self-assessment after the interruption, and then pace your recovery program in keeping with that assessment.

Actively cultivating patience.
Many people feel impatient during the kind of assessment-guided recovery I'm encouraging here. They say

things like, "Why waste time? I'm used to going all-out" or "I feel as if it's a step down if I don't push at my earlier level."

Following a more patient approach isn't always easy. It's normal to want to recover right away. Simply telling yourself to be more patient isn't always enough. To actually become more patient and stay that way, my third guideline is to actively cultivate your patience—in your thoughts, in what you do behaviorally, and in what you focus on when you are doing those behaviors.

In thinking your way to more patience, it's helpful to focus on why you're exercising in the first place. You may have many good reasons, but among them I hope is that you want to have your quality of life be good over the long term. Gradually developed physical fitness is one of the keys to that quality of life. Remind yourself of these reasons whenever as you have impatient thoughts or impulses.

In behaving your way to more patience, first include additional goals for your workout. Then include additional actions to achieve those goals. For example, while gradually recovering her strength and stamina, Clarissa might have chosen to swim shorter distances. The remaining time at the pool could have offered great opportunities for her to pursue an additional goal of improving her basic swimming techniques. It could also have given her time to do some therapeutic stretching, especially beneficial if the improved technique required a greater range of motion. Looking at it more holistically, if she set as one legitimate goal that the whole workout be a mini-vacation from the rest of the day, perhaps she could have included a longer, more relaxed shower after the swim. Any of these activities would have led to achievable benefits, and would have helped her resist burning herself out and giving up.

In focusing your way to more patience, the key ingredient is making truthful, positive comments to yourself on what you are doing during the workout. Examples of truthful, negative comments are, "I'm not swimming as well as I used to" or "Any fool can take an extra long shower!" Examples of truthful, positive comments are, "While I'm gradually working my way back, I'm getting a better chance to work on my technique than when I'm going all out" or "This shower feels good, and I (simply by virtue of being a human being) deserve it!"

Never underestimate the value of positive comments. Positive and negative comments can be equally truthful, but they have opposite effects on how patient you'll be with your recovery program.[15] Honestly acknowledging the negative—preferably with a touch of humor—is fine, but put your emphasis on the positive.

Planning ahead.
Clarissa, like anyone during their first few interruptions, didn't realize how devastating interruptions can be. She wasn't equipped for damage control. Now she can be and

so can you. My fourth guideline, then, has to do with prevention: Whenever possible, anticipate your next interruption, and plan in advance what you'll do to bounce back from it.

Some interruptions are fairly easy to anticipate. For example, vacations and crunches at work often happen on a frequent, if not regular basis. Plan ahead for what you'll do during the interruptions (including having a Plan B) and after the interruption is over (including self-assessing and revising your routine).

For example, if you normally lift weights and are going on a three-week vacation to Mexico, pack some stretch bands for Plan B exercises. Exercise bands don't take up much space. When you return, self-assess and resume with some easy-lift workouts. After that, only gradually increase the weights over the next weeks and months. Your motivation, your fitness program and your elbows, knees, and back will all be better off if you have a careful, pre-planned bounce period as one of your top priorities.

Springboard.

To more easily bounce back from your exercise program's next interruption, consider the following questions. As always, I strongly encourage you to write your answers down and come back to them from time to time for further thought:

1. What do you think will cause your next interruption in your exercise program?
2. When is it likely to occur?
3. What is the best Plan B exercise(s) during the interruption?
4. After the interruption is over:
    a. What can you do to assess your Plan A readiness level?
    b. What specific readjustments are you likely to make in Plan A as a result of your assessment?
    c. How can you actively cultivate your patience during the readjustment period?
        (1) In your thinking (reminders of why)?
        (2) In your behavior (additional goals)?
        (3) In your focus (truthful, positive comments)?

C H A P T E R   8

NO TIME FOR FITNESS?

The Problem: It's about more than time.

A BLUE RIBBON panel could endorse your fitness program, but if you have no time to follow it, your program won't do you any good. Fortunately, your situation may not be totally bleak. Granted, within your current 24/7 week, you may have few discretionary minutes for new activities, but your conclusion that you have zero time for fitness probably hinges on more than that. It's time to look for solutions.

SOLUTIONS

Prioritizing consciously.

Often, statements like "I can't afford X" or "I don't have time for Y" are decisions based on unexamined priorities. Consider some lifestyle differences between Bill and George, two good friends:

Last year, Bill vacationed in Ireland; George bought a new car. Bill says he can't afford a new car; George says he can't afford a vacation in Ireland. When Bill and George are saying what they can and can't afford, are they simply talking about discretionary money or are they also talking about priorities?

Counting shower time, Bill devotes about two hours each day to exercise and George watches television for about two hours each day. Bill says he doesn't have time to watch television; George says he doesn't have time to exercise. When Bill and George are saying what they do and don't have time for, are they talking about their discretionary time or are they also talking about priorities?

Make the activities you do or don't do be options you consciously choose, based on your priorities. Don't be locked into activities you just ended up doing, perhaps at someone else's urging or because you think your friends enjoy them. Make a positive choice to give time to those options that are important to you and choose to minimize the time you give to options that you deem less important. While this is easier to say than to do, it can result in you upgrading your fitness lifestyle.

Examining job demands.
Sometimes prioritizing forces you to look at time-consuming activities you may be uncomfortable even questioning. However, the discomfort may be worth it in the long run.

Let's start with an example my dad told me about. My dad and a man I'll call "Charlie" were foremen in a factory, along with eight other foremen. (This was in the early 1950's, when there were no forewomen in this factory.) Each foreman had a "shop" he was in charge of. Dad worked hard, but when quitting time came, he packed up, and ten minutes later he was usually on his way to play golf (in the early 1950s, playing on public golf courses was less expensive than it is now). Charlie worked hard too, usually staying at least an hour past quitting time. Charlie also worked through most of his breaks, and he often came to work early. The work got done in all of the shops, including Charlie's and Dad's, but the General Foreman—a new guy—was very impressed with Charlie's work ethic.

One day, Dad was out on the factory floor, talking to the General Foreman and the Factory Supervisor, when Charlie went past, almost on the run, doing some errand. When he was out of earshot, the General Foreman began to expound on Charlie's long hours and hard work. Then, with a quick, meaningful glance toward Dad, he said, "This place would really hum if everyone had Charlie's dedication."

My dad's response took the General Foreman by surprise, but had the agreement of the Supervisor:

Dad said, "I don't think so. Actually, as Charlie's boss, I think you have one of two possible problems going on here: On one hand, Charlie may be overworked, in which case you should have another foreman take up some of his responsibilities before he burns out. On the other hand, his workload may be reasonable, but he may not be competent enough to do it in the normal amount of time, in which case you should replace him before he drives his men crazy."

If you don't have time for fitness because your work is too demanding, you might want to think about Charlie and consider the following tough questions:

Are you responsible for an unreasonable amount of work? If so, is this just a temporary situation or is it permanent? It's permanent for a lot of people. If it's permanent for you, how long do you plan to tolerate it? You may not think you have much of a choice in the matter, especially if you've been led to expect "real" choices to be comfortable and simple, between purely "good" alternatives (i.e., with no negatives included) and purely "bad" ones (i.e., with no positives included). With many overly demanding jobs, neither staying nor leaving is a "pure" alternative. Each is likely to involve mixtures of positives and negatives. I hope you'll think through those mixtures before you choose to leave or to continue staying. I'll leave it up to the rest of society to give you arguments in favor of staying. In contrast, I'd suggest that if you consider the hazards to your physical and mental health and the impact on the people you care most about, not to mention your fitness, you may conclude that at some point a job change is a bargain, even if it involves a cut in pay.

Is your job over your head? If so, is this just temporary, as is often the case when someone is given a new responsibility, or is it permanent? Is it a matter of just getting up to speed, or is it a matter of being under-qualified and always having to overcompensate because of a bad person-to-job match-up? If it's the latter, the glamour of your job will wear off and I would encourage you to seek a better match-up as soon as possible.

Are you tied to a job that is too demanding because you are supporting a lifestyle—yours or that of a significant other— that's too expensive? Ah, life's layers of complexity! While some of the "best things in life are free," some nice (but not necessary) things in life are not free. If you have possessions, activities or people in your life that are costing you too much for the benefits they give you—especially after you are worn out from an overly demanding job that they require you to keep—consider simplifying your life. In terms of quality and quantity of life, more than fitness may be at stake.

Can you do some fitness activity each day (regardless of your answers to the above questions)? Most people, no matter what else they do, have 15 or 20 minutes a day that could have gone to exercise. For example, Tony, an attorney, bikes on the weekends, both for fitness and recreation. However, during the work-week, his large blocks of time go to his profession and to his family, and not to exercise. Instead, he creates a number of small blocks for exercise, usually between clients. These blocks include going up and down several flights of stairs and doing 10 or 15 weight reps—all in less than 10 minutes while listening to top-of-the-hour news. He finds these exercise breaks refreshing and beneficial to his work. Also, when driving would only be five minutes faster than walking to lunches, meetings or court, he walks.

If you don't have even 15 or 20 minutes, maybe you can do things like use the stairs instead of the elevator, or park further away from your job so that you walk an extra five minutes each way. Use your time limitation as a frame within which to be creative. The benefits may not happen as quickly as when you spend more time, but some of them still can happen. Something is better than nothing.

Overcoming the discomfort of change.
Lack of time is often the reason people give when their deeper problem is actually a discomfort with change. The thought of change can seem so overwhelming that the cost of whatever time it takes to make the change seems prohibitive. Some people have more tolerance for change than others, but for any of us there is some level of change that we will resist, even if the benefits are overwhelmingly obvious.

I witnessed this one time at a wellness conference: The conference went for five days. The setting was a college campus during a summer break. Nearly two hundred health professionals ate and slept in one of the college's residence halls. The conference organizers collaborated with the caterers to insure that all of our food was at the highest level of nutrition and intended for health enhancement. Salt and animal fat were at a minimum; whole grains, fresh fruit (especially blue-berries and melons) and fresh vegetables were abundant. All the desserts, while delicious, were from "healthy," low calorie recipes.

The first evening after arrival, the conference participants raved about this wonderful food selection. I heard a lot of people say things like, "If only people could eat like this all the time!" I heard similar comments at breakfast and lunch the following day. Interestingly, the praises began to trail off a bit by evening of the second day. They became non-existent by the evening of the third day. On the evening of the fourth day, a "revolt" occurred. That is, a large contingent of the conference participants skipped the "wonderful" supper and instead opted for cheeseburgers and fries at a nearby fast-food restaurant.

Mind you, these weren't ordinary people. Rather, their specialized training made them unusually conscious of the benefits of healthy eating. Their own personal diets were already better than the norm, and they spent a lot of their professional time encouraging others to eat better. Nevertheless, they found the change from (some) junk food in their lives to 100% healthy eating to be too radical.

Whatever level of change is too radical for you, once you reach it, anything more will be unpleasant and something you will seek to avoid. A key concern with potential change can be the pressure—often well intended—that others put on you. For example, suppose you jog several times a week and would enjoy jogging with a friend who jogs every day, but in contrast to your friend, you don't want to jog every day. Or maybe you'd like to play basketball a couple of evenings each week, but don't want to make the time commitment you'd need to make if you joined the league team your buddies play on. In either case, you might be tempted to say, "I can't," and perhaps you might even arrange things in other parts of your life to make that statement seem true. Unfortunately, this approach may cut you off from those times when you do want to jog with your friend or play basketball with your buddies. Before deciding what to say to others, and especially before saying "I can't," consider the following steps for a more comfortable and more rewarding approach to change:

Respect your present tolerance level. Whether your personal tolerance for change is high or low, it probably developed out of a combination of inherited tendencies and accumulated life experiences. You probably didn't develop it overnight, so you can't expect to alter it overnight either. Rather than try to alter it drastically, I'd suggest that you consider the possibility that for many parts of your life, your tolerance level is fine the way it is. Instead, at least for achieving your goal of developing a higher fitness level, recognize your present tolerance level and introduce changes gradually. Using the above examples, maybe you'd find it most comfortable to start jogging with your friend on only one specified day per week, jogging alone on any other day, and seeing how that goes before making a larger commitment. Similarly, maybe you'd be most comfortable starting with the league team as an alternate, rather than as a regular team member.

Own the activity.[16] No one wants to be forced or manipulated into a fitness level. If someone else's reasons for you to get more involved overlap with your own, that's fine, as long as your focus is on your reasons. Keeping the focus on your reasons will help you keep their "support" from being a "control" to revolt against. When it comes to exercise, probably no one has time to be controlled by someone else, but most of us have time to revolt, possibly by saying, "I don't have time."

When owning the activity, never make your commitment with a "Do I have to?" attitude. If you decide to jog with a friend once a week (instead of seven times as she'd prefer) or if you decide to be on a league team only as an alternate, make sure you are making this commitment for your reasons and then take it on enthusiastically. Otherwise you risk dooming the whole endeavor to failure, not to mention being a "wet blanket."

Demand your right to imperfection. In many ways, our society demands perfection. But one of the best ways to undermine anything is to demand that it be perfect. With this demand, anything less than perfect will feel like a failure. Setting yourself up for failure is not very motivating. On the other hand, if you demand the right to imperfection, you can't lose! You've allowed room for improvement, an ironically optimistic stance.

Often a major problem that accompanies demands for perfection is an unwritten rule that makes any deviation from one's commitment seem almost like a mortal sin. Some days you are going to be too sick to jog with your friend or to be an alternate on the league team. Also sometimes another responsibility is going to legitimately take higher priority. If change requires an unduly rigid follow-through on your commitment, who wouldn't have a low tolerance for change? So along with demanding the right to imperfection, demand reasonable flexibility.

Work through the change ahead of time. While the purpose of making any change is to get something that is desirable (in this case, fun and increased fitness), one of the scariest things about anything new is the possibility that it will trigger something that is undesirable. Remember that your present lifestyle already has a structure to it, one that may be affected by the change. You may make a change and find that some other activities have to be rescheduled or dropped, and you may have to deal with other people's feelings about these changes. If you work through the likely problems ahead of time, the main change isn't going to loom as threatening when it is time to make it.

Overcoming energy problems.
Just as when people feel overwhelmed by the prospect of change, when they feel too tired to break with an old routine or to initiate a new vigorous activity, they often feel

as if they don't have time to do it. In such cases, addressing the energy issues may be more helpful than trying to find more time.

Check with your doctor. We all have our ups and downs, and you may think your occasional "downs" are normal. On the other hand, if they are severe or if you're almost always down—too "down" to feel like doing anything active—don't simply shrug it off as normal. Something might be wrong. Among the many possibilities, you might have a sleep disorder, iron deficiency anemia, a hormone deficiency, or you might be depressed. (In the case of depression, you might be surprised to hear your doctor confirm your intentions to exercise, since exercise is often one of the more effective ways to treat certain depressions.) Whatever the possibility, you should consult with your physician. These and many other problems can be treated. Fitness concerns aside, your overall quality of life and quantity of life may be at stake.

Consider your biorhythms. Let's suppose the physician gives you a clean bill of health, but you still lack energy. Perhaps the next thing to consider is when you lack energy. Our biological levels rise and fall throughout the day, causing us to feel energetic sometimes and sluggish at other times. If we get enough sleep and if we go to bed and get up at fairly consistent times, our biological patterns become consistent, too. When this happens, we can predict when we're likely to feel most energetic and most sluggish. Perhaps you have tried to do your exercise at one of your metabolic low points and simply need to reschedule it to one of your "prime" times. On the other hand, perhaps your sleep times are so variable that your body has neither an established rhythm nor a predictable "prime time."

Here, establishing a rhythm is your first step. Depending on how variable your present sleep times are, this may take more than just a couple days of consistent routine. Be patient with yourself as you create the necessary structure to make a new routine comfortable and automatic.

Employ warm-up activities. Some people are "slow starters" when it comes to exercise. Once their muscles (and perhaps their brains) are warmed up, they do fine, but until then, they feel sluggish. If you are unclear on how to create a good warm-up routine, consult with a personal trainer. Along with warming you up and helping you get started, your routine can help you loosen up your muscles, perhaps preventing an injury.

Distinguish between emotional energy and physical energy. Have you ever had a time after a day at your job or caring for a child when you felt drained of energy, but then had to do a prolonged physical activity and ended up feeling fine? Think of the low energy you initially felt as a drain of "emotional energy" rather than of "physical energy." The tiredness can feel the same either way, pleading with you, saying, "Do nothing! No exertion, please!"

The bad news is that if you are having an emotional energy drain at workout time, your tiredness is giving you the wrong message. Obeying it by being sedentary may cause you to skip your exercise. The good news is that if—with only a little discomfort—you put the tiredness message on hold and gently begin to exercise, you will be able to soon tell whether you're dealing with an emotional drain or a physical drain. Continued fatigue after ten or fifteen minutes of moderately vigorous activity would suggest that you are having a physical drain and you should stop for the day. On the other hand, if you feel yourself starting to perk up and feel refreshed after that ten or fifteen minutes, you're probably starting to recover from an emotional drain, in which case you more likely should continue the workout. Emotional refreshment at the cost of some moderate physical exertion is a pretty good bargain.

Managing Daily Interruptions.
People in all walks of life get interrupted. Whether you are a lawyer, a professor, an entrepreneur, or the parent at home with a colicky baby, not all of your interruptions can be (nor should be) eliminated. If an interruption involves something both important and urgent, you should stop what you are doing and respond to the interruption right away. But many interruptions are better thought of as interferences—interferences to be dealt with later, if at all.

Paula's situation provides a good example. She was a new Residence Hall Supervisor at a large university. She was also a graduate student in Higher Education and a long-time jogger. From the start, the nature of her job seemed designed to take its toll on both her studies and her fitness. While it didn't help that she had unlimited access to all the dorm food she could possibly eat, her main problem was the frequent interruptions brought on by her job.

Any crisis or disruption within the university's Housing Division called for an impromptu meeting of supervisors and upper level Housing administrators. Worse still, her job required her to be available most hours of most days for residents or Resident Advisors in her dorm that wanted her help. The evenings, nights and weekends were no better than the weekdays because they allowed students more time to get into mischief or seek a captive audience to hear their grievances when their boyfriends or girlfriends broke up with them.

If she added up the free minutes in her day, Paula had time, but finding predictable blocks of time to study seemed impossible. Also there never seemed to be a block of time she could depend on for a jog, and her boss looked askance at time away from the dorm, unless for classes or meetings. By the end of Paula's first month on the job, she was behind in most of her classes and she was getting soft. In fact, to her dismay, she realized that she had already gained five pounds. If she wasn't careful, she'd have a new body by the end of the school year, one she didn't prefer over her present one.

Her employment contract went for the entire school year and she needed the money. She felt that the experiences gained from being a Residence Hall Supervisor could enhance her future career, so she didn't want to leave her job if she didn't have to. On the other hand, letting her job make her so vulnerable to interruptions was sabotaging progress toward her long-term goals. She had to find different ways to do her job.

By now, she was already familiar with the nature of her interruptions, but for the first time she thought about the patterns of her interruptions. She realized there was a block from noon to 1:30 p.m. that was almost always free of interruptions. Apparently, students either stayed on campus over the noon hour or were in too much of a hurry to get back to classes after lunch to stop to see her. Also, her bosses, busy with lunch meetings, never called their impromptu staff meetings during that time period. This could be a good opportunity for Paula to work on projects requiring blocks of time.

When she thought about the various physical and psychological emergencies residents came to her with, she acknowledged that she would always want to respond to these. Sometimes they occurred well into the night. However, she realized that she never once had a call or a knock on her door early in the mornings. Some of her fellow supervisors had developed irregular sleep patterns, the result of sleeping in after late night emergencies. She could avoid that cycle by always getting up at 7 o'clock, no matter what time she went to bed, and using the next hour for jogging. If she needed to take one or two cat-naps later in the day, she would, but the jogging was going to happen. For the remote possibility of an early morning emergency, she carried her cell phone with her on her jog.

Finally, Paula had received complaints from the dorm study hall, which operated from 7 to 11 p.m. each evening; some residents were making too much noise, distracting others who came there to get things done. Was she ever happy to begin personally monitoring that problem! She brought in a larger desk, put a "Residence Hall Supervisor" sign on it, and established order in a way that would have amazed the strictest of high school study hall monitors. The students who wanted to study loved this change, and voted positively for it with their feet. Any resident or Resident Advisor could still ask her to step outside and talk if they really needed something, but they now went elsewhere if they simply wanted a lone-liness fix or someone to procrastinate with.

These changes marked the beginning of Paula's return to good academic standing and fitness. Meanwhile, her boss was impressed.

Understanding the pattern of her interruptions and being creative were all Paula needed to get her life back on track. Similarly, professors, after analyzing the patterns of interruptions by students, often designate certain time periods as weekly "office hours" and use others as times to work in a library carrel, disappearing among rows of books. Likewise, entrepreneurs, after identifying the pattern and nature of client and salesperson interruptions, train subordinates to handle certain categories of problems, referring only the delicate concerns to "the boss." Even if there seems to be no pattern, as might be the case facing the parent of a colicky baby, knowing that fact and understanding the nature of the baby's problems might help the parent more intelligently do things like setting up a babysitting pool with other parents or rearranging alternate workout times with his/her partner.

The following steps can help you address interruptions in your life:

First, don't plan to get rid of all your interruptions; some should stay—those that are both important and urgent.[17]

Second, study the nature and patterns of your interruptions with the help of a written record. This may need to be fairly detailed to find your time leaks.

Third, set up a structure that (a) allows the important-and-urgent interruptions to reach you, while it also (b) protects you from the other ones, at least while you are doing your higher priority activities.

Springboard.

Along with my recommendations, I've asked some uncomfortable questions in this chapter. I hope I won't seem too obnoxious if I finish up with two more:

First, have you ever wondered whether you were fooling yourself with your reasons?

And second, have you ever wondered whether your "lack of time" arguments were just bogus excuses to stay put?

These are tough questions, especially since some rare people really don't have the time. If you think that's you, no doubt you would like assurance that you didn't just make it up. You'd like to think you were looking objectively at all the facts, and not just presenting things in a way to favor your short-term comforts or whatever.

If you're haunted by this kind of doubt, here's a quick test that might give you some clarity. I call it The Million Dollars Test. It helps detect con-jobs people do on themselves. It has just three questions:

First, if someone offered you a million dollars to design and follow-through on a fitness lifestyle for yourself, starting next week, could you do it?

Second, would the resulting quality/quantity of life be worth at least a million dollars?

and

Third, for which of your future days are the first two questions irrelevant?

If you answered, "yes" to the first two questions and "none" to the third, I hope you'll resume your search for more solutions and not give in to your time limitations. Your quality of life—and possibly the quality for those you care about—may depend on it.

C H A P T E R   9

PHYSICAL LIMITATIONS

The Problem: Choosing realistic goals.

WHETHER YOU ARE elderly, chronically ill, overweight, classified as handicapped, an average "Joe" or "Jill," or a reigning Olympic champion, placing unduly low or unduly high expectations on yourself can lead to poor motivation for fitness activities. The converse is also true: assuming a favorable benefit/cost ratio, if you define success in terms of goals and sub-goals which are personally challenging but achievable, you can have great motivation for physical exercise regardless of age or circumstance. Choosing realistic goals is a core principle through this *Guide*. It merits extra discussion when addressing physical limitations, since these "limitations" often, but not always, reduce one's range of realistic goals.

SOLUTIONS

Seeking professional advice.

One day in the locker room, after a hard workout, a friend of mine slapped his work-out partner on the back

111

and said, "Man, we really kicked butt today!" His friend responded, "Well, like ole Nietzsche used to say, 'That which doesn't kill me makes me stronger!'" A newcomer interrupted this celebration saying, "Yeah, but how do you know which it's gonna be?"

The new guy had asked a reasonable question. Even for already active people, once their bodies have aged enough to become less predictable, it's reasonable to wonder. For people who have never been active or who have acquired certain physical limitations, it's both a reasonable and a frequent concern.[18]

How do you know if everything is all right when you have physiological reactions to vigorous activity? What if your body's reactions are warning signals of impending doom? Is it good that you're breathing hard, or that your heart rate is elevated, or that your arms or legs feel heavy? Which reactions should you be afraid of? Will your exertions trigger a heart attack or will they lead to better health and well-being?

With doubts about what is safe, many people decide against exercise. Unfortunately, that decision, in the long term, can lead them to more severe physical limitations. Instead, consider easing your concerns by consulting with relevant professionals. Start by getting a medical clearance from a physician who specializes in your area of concern. Then, seek up-to-date information from a combination of professionals about what kinds of exercise are safe for you. Also get recommendations on a safe starting level, and a safe path of progression from that level to one that will give you a satisfactory fitness enhancing effect.[19] Start with the physician who cleared you, possibly later collaborating with a physical therapist or a personal trainer. Along with increasing your safety, these consultations can help you avoid other injury-causing, motivation-killing mistakes, and put you on a good path toward fitness.

Questioning "can't do."
Whatever your ability level, if you want to improve it, avoid spending too much time doing workouts that are boringly easy. Concomitantly, avoid spending time doing workouts that are impossibly difficult. The first extreme will have you quitting out of a sense of meaninglessness while the second will have you quitting out of a sense of despair. This means that you have to find out what you can do and what you can't do.

However, using the term "can't do" can cause problems. After the various failures and setbacks that anyone has had by the time they reach adulthood, "can't do" comes to mean something more permanent than it should. It definitely comes to mean something different than "currently unable to do." No matter who you are or what your physical circumstances happen to be, there are things you "can't do" and indeed may never be able to do. At the same time, by overusing the phrase, you run the risk of closing yourself off from other things you are only unable to do currently.

If you are going to overuse one phrase or the other, I'd suggest it be the phrase "currently unable to do." That phrase puts your focus on what you currently can do, and lets you build from there. The mantra's long version might be something like, "Despite my current limitation X, I still can do activity Y, so that's what I'm going to do for now." Sometimes "current limitation X" will actually prove to be permanent, but other times it may prove to have been only temporary.

John's story provides a good case in point: John was a retired English professor. After his annual physical, his doctor warned him that his excess weight and family history put him at risk for diabetes and heart disease.

John promptly consulted a nutritionist and soon made a successful transition to a much-improved diet. Unfortunately, his weight did not drop enough. His nutritionist advised him to consult with a personal trainer and add exercise to his lifestyle.

The personal trainer suggested a routine of daily walks with weight training three times a week. One purpose of the weight training was to increase John's muscle mass. The additional muscle mass would burn up calories that otherwise helped maintain John's fat. The strategy made sense to John, but he had some concerns.

"I've never been very active," he explained. "I've always been weak, so I put my energies into my books.

I'll try the walking, but I don't think I can do the weights."

His trainer smiled. "You know, I have a couple of my clients do five push-ups every time they say, 'I can't.'"

"Why do you do that?" John asked. "Besides, I can't do one push-up, let alone five!"

"Oops! There you did it again," his trainer laughed. "My purpose isn't to punish people who use the 'c-word,' but rather to remind them to put their focus on what they are able to do, and build from there. If you focus on what you can't do, you may never accomplish anything."

From there, the trainer assessed what John was currently able to do, and prescribed a program that started at that level. He increased the level only as John's strength increased. At first, none of the weights were even as heavy as a gallon of milk.

By the time John had completed the first year of his combined diet-exercise program, he felt much better and he was on a slow, steady trend of weight loss. Now he could easily do the five push-ups if the trainer heard him say, "I can't"—but that never happened.

The basic strategy for increasing John's abilities would be the same if he were a partially paralyzed thirty-year old, or an Olympic figure skater in her teens. No matter who you are or what your physical circumstances are, putting your focus on what you can't do hinders you. Instead, identify your present ability level and then look for the most helpful things you can do to work up from that level.

Embracing Path B.

Sometimes focusing on what you can do actually does require you to go in a completely different direction than you've gone in the past or would initially prefer to go. Let's call your preferred direction "Path A." If Path A is clearly closed off to you, focusing on what you still can do may mean looking for a Path B. Unfortunately, getting enthusiastic about Path B can be hard if you haven't let go of Path A.

Let me illustrate this with an easy, *non*-fitness example: I love apples. As I think of how I enjoy a fresh apple's sweetness and crunchiness and juiciness and even its tartness, my mouth waters. On the other hand, I love apple pie too.

One morning, my wife, Carolyn, told me she wanted to bake an apple pie. All day at work I looked forward to eating apple pie and ice cream. When I got home that evening, I opened the door and breathed in, smelling for the pie, but it hadn't been baked. Some unexpected things had taken up Carolyn's day, and she barely had time to buy the apples, let alone make the pie. Seeing the look on my face, she laughed and jokingly said, "Oh well, at least we have the apples. Here—you like apples. Have one!" Recognizing that she was serious, I obediently took a bite.

Now here is the interesting part: With my mind still locked in on apple pie and ice cream, the mere apple may as well have been a raw potato for all the enjoyment

I got from it. Only after I let go of the pie idea and started tasting for the apple could I again enjoy the apple's sweetness, crunch, juiciness and tartness.

Obviously, a lot of things in life are harder to let go of than apple pie, but the principle remains the same. You can't get the full value out of Path B if you haven't yet let go of Path A.

When it is hard to let go of Path A, as is often the case when you encounter a serious physical setback, at least two processes may be at work and each may need some time. The first is the process of recognizing with both your head and your heart that Path A is no longer an option for you. Your head (your intellect) may catch on right away, but it may take your heart (your emotional attachments, values, hopes, fantasies, etc.) a bit longer. Be patient as you let your head "talk" to your heart.

Before the heart grasps the point, it first may have to "grieve" the loss of Path A. Especially, it may have to come to terms with memories and dashed expectations tied to various things in your life that somehow tie in with your (in)ability to pursue Path A. Of course, this grieving, while normal, can be painful.

You may find that this grieving has similarities with other losses you've experienced, losses not related to physical limitations. For example, suppose you've had to go through the unwanted break-up of a long-term romantic relationship. At first, when things like certain songs or places reminded you of your ex-lover, the feelings of loss were acute, even if the rest of your day had been relatively normal. Slowly, as your heart painfully worked through the feelings triggered by these things (the songs, places, etc.), those feelings, while not necessarily "happy," at least became more neutral.

A person recovering from an injury that permanently deprives him/her of an exercise-related Path A may face something similar. Consider, for example, a (now) ex-runner who feels loss when seeing a group of joggers go down the street or hearing a couple friends talking about their most recent 10K. Before feeling much enthusiasm for swimming or some other perfectly good Path B, the ex-runner's heart may first have to work through feelings of loss triggered by those Path A-related situations.

As with any grieving, let it happen at its own pace. Don't torture yourself by trying to put the various sensitive situations under a microscope and looking at them all the time; and don't try to always shove the situations or feelings under the rug when you encounter them. Eventually, as your head and heart deal with the various ways you feel the losses, the losses will hit you with less force and frequency. Then you can develop more enthusiasm for Path B. At any time during the grief process, but especially if the healing trend doesn't seem to be developing, please seek the help of a professional counselor.

Remember, you can recover. Here are two quite different examples of successful recovery:

Chris is a 35 year-old man who is a very good wheelchair racer. Once he was an excellent high school runner who planned on running for many years to come. Then he permanently lost the use of his legs in a car accident. As part of his psychological recovery, he had to go through the process of letting go of running. Once that was accomplished, he embraced wheelchair racing. Over the years, he's stayed very fit, and he's found this second pastime very satisfying.

Tim and several buddies jogged together at noon each day for many years. Then, in his mid-fifties, Tim developed severe degenerative arthritis in the ball of his right foot, apparently stemming from an injury he'd suffered years earlier. Now, bouncing off that foot hurt too much to make jogging a reasonable option. Giving up jogging meant giving up a satisfying social activity as well as a satisfying physical activity. At first that was difficult. Eventually, he realized that while he had to give up jogging, he didn't have to give up his friends or fitness. Now he has coffee with his buddies. He bikes for fitness. He enjoys both activities.

I'm sure you can come up with similar examples, and in each case I'd bet that the person had to let go of Path A before he/she could embrace Path B.

Doing Path A differently.
Sometimes Path A isn't the problem as much as is the way you travel on it. Jesse didn't need to let go of Path A, but he did have to let go of some unrealistic goals:

In his teens and early twenties, Jesse was a good, all-around athlete. Over the years, he stayed fit through cross-training. In a typical week, he would swim two days with his wife, lift weights two days with several friends, and bike two days by himself. Also, almost every day he took a walk in the evening with his wife. This routine worked well for him, not only in terms of fitness, but also in meeting his social and psychological needs. The swimming and the walks were something special between him and his wife, the weight lifting was a fun, "guy thing," and the bike workouts gave him some "alone time" which he also needed.

Then, in his late 50's, Jesse took the wrong slant on things after reading a newspaper article about a man 25 years older than himself. This man looked much younger than his actual age. Also, despite the fact that he was about Jesse's size, this man could bench press 50 pounds more than Jesse could! For over 30 years, Jesse and his lifting buddies had managed to focus on fairly non-competitive personal goals and to support each others' efforts. For over 30 years, no one got injured, they had fun and they all benefited. Somehow, though, this article awakened a mindset within Jesse which had been dormant since his early teens: "I'll be damned if some guy in his 80's is going to out-lift me!"

With this change, Jesse stepped up his weight lifting with the goal of overtaking the older man. Contrary to his friends' advice, he pushed his limits relentlessly, especially on the bench press. Nevertheless, progress was minimal—not surprising, since years of lifting already had him near the upper end of his natural ability range.

With his unrealistic goals, workouts became less fun. Before long he found himself with a severely injured right shoulder.

For a while, the injury cast a negative shadow over his entire cross training program—shoulders are a part of swimming and biking too, and his wife didn't particularly like to hear him obsessing over his injury on their walks.

Finally, Dan, one of the guys in Jesse's lifting group, set him straight: "Look Jesse, I can't out-lift that old man either. Does that make me a loser in your eyes?"

"No."

"Then how special do you think you are that you're a loser if you can't out-lift him? Maybe he has more ability than both of us put together. Does that make him a better person? Does it mean we should just up-and-quit? You've been doing great for years, but lately you're putting your ego into this stuff and acting stupid! What's wrong with just keeping fit and enjoying life like you used to?"

Jesse didn't exactly give Dan a standing ovation for this speech, but the message got through, and after a couple months of physical therapy on his shoulder, Jesse worked his way back into the old routine.

It's possible that there is a bit of Jesse in all of us. If that's the case, I hope we'll all have a voice like Dan's in our lives to set us straight when our egos clash with our limitations, and when we forget why we are exercising in the first place.

Working with others.

Some people have training partners. Others join water aerobics classes, Zumba classes, yoga classes, martial arts clubs, running clubs, or other groups. They do so because the members learn from each other, they get realistic inspiration and incentives from each other, they provide structure for each other, and they have fun. These people don't have an exclusive right to such benefits. The benefits can be there for you, too. Lists of local clubs and classes relevant to your interests and limitations are available at many fitness centers, hospitals, clinics and rehabilitation facilities. If you don't feel compatible with the groups in your area, the internet can help you connect with people from organizations further away who can advise you on how to form your own group. Remember, you aren't under a sentence to always have to go it alone. Forming or joining a group can be well worth your effort.[20]

An apology.

I am an optimistic person. I hope you'll think of me as a realistically optimistic person. Either way, I hope my optimism and enthusiasm don't come off as a lack of appreciation for how difficult it can be for you to overcome a physical limitation and succeed in following a fitness lifestyle.

If in any way I have seemed to belittle or trivialize what you are up against, please accept my sincere apology. In no way do I think it is easy to overcome a physical limitation. Using the lingo of this *Guide,* I appreciate the fact that you may be having to adjust to goals and expectations in ways you might not have preferred. You may be facing quite large "costs" for the benefits of a fitness lifestyle. I only hope that the material I offer helps you accept those new goals and expectations and offset the costs with even larger benefits.

Springboard.

Except for putting additional focus on what you can do currently, and building from there, the following steps are basically the same as in the Springboard for Chapter Three:

1. Carefully choose the type of fitness activity you'll be doing:
   a. Write down what fitness benefits you most want.
   b. List all of the types of activities that might give you these benefits. Include those that you currently can do at some level. Don't be afraid to include some which are beyond what you currently can do.
   c. Consult with a physician, physical therapist and/or personal trainer who specializes in your area of concern for ideas, including on:
      (1) Possible additions to the list of activities,

(2) The likely costs for each activity.

(3) Alternatives for those activities whose costs will be too high or benefits too low.

(4) Alternatives for activities when your chances of a satisfying level of success are low.

d. Modify your list of fitness activities to try, based on likely cost/benefit ratios and chances for success.

e. Finally, choose among the remaining alternatives, based on your personal likes and dislikes.

2. Preferably with the help of a physical therapist or personal trainer, choose a convenient time and place for your fitness activity, work from within your current ability range, and organize your activity so that each time you do it, the benefits you feel (such as enjoyments, satisfactions or feelings of accomplishment) outweigh any of its costs (including lingering fatigue). Keeping a workout log can help you make fair assessments of ongoing costs and benefits and help monitor your progress.

3. Address the issue of reasonable expectations:

a. Injuries lower your chances of success. You can prevent many injuries by consulting with experts on such things as proper equipment, (including basic running or walking shoes), and proper technique (for walking, running, etc., but especially for weight lifting). [NOTE: This is not where you should try to get by cheaply. Any sweatshirt or tee shirt will do the job, but check references, not merely prices, in selecting a doctor or trainer or buying equipment, even shoes.]

b. Structure your program so that, as you progress from one level of difficulty to the next, you can reasonably expect success within a relatively short period of time at the new level.

c. At the beginning of any next higher level, if you are not sure how much to challenge yourself, err on the light side and see how you feel over the following few days. If you find yourself unduly tired or sore, go lighter still until your body starts to adjust.

d. Only after your body seems to have adjusted should you gradually increase the challenge beyond your present level.

e. Don't worry if your increases in activity are slower or smaller than someone else's. Another person's more rapid increases in activity may contribute to their quitting later on. At any rate, you aren't in a contest or up against a deadline. Rather, you are trying to develop a personal fitness program that will last.

4. Give your program a fair try. This especially includes consulting with professionals if you

encounter difficulties. Let them help you make appropriate adjustments. Don't let misguided machoism or a sense of shame tempt you to quit instead of telling them what they need to know to help you.

5. Assess your reactions. Keep a log. Note changes in your motivation. Note lapses in your exercise routine. Ask yourself what's going on. Look for patterns. Identify triggers. Experiment. Be a detective!

SOCIAL OBSTACLES

The Problem: Other people "misbehave."

WHETHER YOU THINK of social obstacles as "costs" or as factors that lower your expectations of success, they can place a heavy toll on your motivation. (Here, we're focusing on motivation to seek fitness, though you'll quickly recognize that learning to overcome social obstacles can be relevant for many parts of your life.) Beyond interfering with motivation, social obstacles can block any number of seemingly reasonable plans for transforming your motivations into a fitness lifestyle. Very likely the people who put up these obstacles are people you know rather than strangers. Obviously this can make your problem more difficult. When it is a stranger, maybe the guy who yells at you from his car as you jog down the street or the one who ogles you at the gym, you can usually fix the problem by doing something simple like changing your jogging route or by exercising in the screened area of the gym. The problem is more difficult to solve when the obstacles come from someone you know, someone you may have to deal with frequently, and possibly someone you care about.

It isn't always easy when your spouse objects to changes in the foods you want to serve or be served. Also, it isn't easy when your in-laws make fun of your fitness activities or seem suspicious of your motives—e.g., "Who do you have in mind that you want to look so good for?" And it isn't easy when roommates or friends from the office badger you to do things with them when you want to exercise, and seem to feel hurt or angry when you turn them down.

Let's use "misbehave" as a fairly neutral term to cover all the ways other people interfere with, undermine, or discourage you in your fitness efforts. This chapter offers strategies for understanding and coping with other people's misbehaviors.

Consider what may cause people to put up the obstacles. Despite their obnoxious impact, they are probably responding to some very normal, human concerns. Unless you know what those concerns are, you are likely to begin thinking of these people as immature, sick, or sinister. Occasionally you will be right, but often you won't be. Either way, your views won't necessarily stop them from interfering with the quality of your fitness lifestyle. Two types of factors may be causing their misbehaviors.

First, people misbehave when they are in "pain." Let's use "pain" to cover the many possible psychological discomforts (such as feelings of sadness, stresses, insecurities or threats) as well as many possible physical discomforts (such as aches, feelings of fatigue and illness) that can push a person to misbehave toward you. While some misbehaviors may strike you as outrageous, you may consider others more forgivable once you understand the person's pain.

Here are some examples of people misbehaving in response to pain:

Adrian and Megan have been married for ten years. Both are in their early thirties, they enjoy their careers, and they have no desire to have children. In their teens, and early twenties, each was active and lean. Over the past five or six years each has become more sedentary, and each seems on a significant trend of gaining weight.

Adrian comes from a family of large people and views the weight gains as a normal, even healthy process. Not so for Megan, who comes from a family of fitness enthusiasts. Megan's recent alarm over her weight gains and her desire to get fit again seem alien to Adrian. For him, everything was fine the way it was, and now Megan is spoiling it. For him, the only explanation that makes sense goes back to a painful period during their engagement when she had a brief fling with one of her co-workers. He wonders if she has developed a wandering eye again and fears dark motives with her "fitness kick." As a result, he continually schedules them both for other things during Megan's exercise times, he often sulks before and after she goes to the gym, and he suggests eating out or frequently brings home "treats" of ice cream, chocolates and her favorite pastries.

Ron and Jan are the parents of three very energetic young children, the oldest five years of age. Ron is a young professional, working hard to get established in his company. Jan, for these years, is a stay-at-home mom. By evening each day, she is worn to a frazzle. Feeling lonely and hoping for some help with the kids while she prepares supper, Jan looks forward to Ron's arrival home each evening.

Recently, Ron came home and enthusiastically told Jan that he wanted to enroll in his company's fitness program; it goes for an hour each day, right after work. To his surprise, Jan burst into tears, screamed, "I hate you!" and stormed out of the room. Since then Jan has refused to talk about exercise. When he tries to talk about it, she says, "You do whatever you want," and gives him the cold shoulder. Since Ron and Jan were both active before they had kids, Ron feels confused by what to him seems to be a reversal on her part.

None of us are mind readers. Even when we are aware of some of the pains another person is feeling, we are usually more aware of our own concerns and of the misbehavior the other person is inflicting on us. Our tendency is to respond sharply to the misbehaviors or to withdraw. Doing either of these can intensify the other person's pain, and possibly intensify his/her misbehavior.

The first communication approach I'll describe, assertive communication, will instead have you explore for a better remedy with the other person. Ideally, this approach will help you both discuss the pain, help you to make a humane contact with the other person's pain (sometimes that's the main thing needed), and then more effectively help the two of you address the misbehavior.

However, before I discuss assertive communication, consider also the other main cause for the misbehaviors we're concerned with: People misbehave when they've learned the wrong thing or haven't learned the right thing. With the two preceding examples, I focused on "misbehaviors" of spouses in response to pain. You could also argue that with each couple, the other spouse was "misbehaving" too, not necessarily in response to pain as much as in response to poor previous learning experiences—experiences that taught them to focus too much on their own agendas or not enough on the other person's. Megan, the wife in the first example, failed to think in advance about Adrian's concerns despite her knowledge of his family's values and of the mistrust she generated in the past. Ron, the husband in the second example, failed to consider the impact of a late afternoon exercise routine on his frazzled wife or on his children. Instead, both Megan and Ron only focused on what they wanted to do. We will hope that both learn from their present experiences.

Meanwhile, Howard provides another example of a person misbehaving, also in part as a function of having learned to do the wrong thing or not to do the right thing: When Howard was in sixth grade, he and his male classmates ran after the girls they liked, trying to pull their pony-tails or steal their caps. The girls would squeal and retaliate, everyone would laugh, and to Howard it seemed like a good time. Soon enough the other guys learned better ways to get the girls' attentions, but for some reason Howard never did.

Of course, as an adult, Howard doesn't pull pony-tails or run off with women's caps, but he teases in ways that are unwanted and aggravating. Typically, the women he teases feel trapped. They may give mild protests, but mainly they half-giggle, blush, look down, and pray for someone else to change the topic. Afterwards, of course, they avoid Howard as much as possible, but their earlier smiles, giggles and blushes encourage Howard to bother them some more.

Ann, who lives in the apartment next to Howard, has come to dread seeing him when she leaves or returns in her workout clothes. Much more often than would happen by chance, Howard will pop out, ready to comment on her fitness progress. His leers make Ann want to apologize for wearing ordinary active wear and trying to be anything other than sedentary. Being sedentary isn't very appealing to Ann, but being leered at is worse. Lately she has found herself staying inside more, skipping workouts. She feels stuck, at least until her lease expires.

Just as one doesn't have to be a bad person to feel pain, one doesn't have to be a bad person to have learned the wrong thing or to have not learned the right thing. Recognizing that every person feels some sort of pain, and that every person has some "mis-learning," may help you respond more gently and effectively.

SOLUTIONS

Communicating assertively.[21]

If you want to take care of yourself, you'll want the misbehavior to stop. If you want to maintain the relationship, and especially if you have positive attachment to the person doing the misbehavior, you'll also want to take care of the other person, and possibly that person's pain or mis-education. With assertive communication you can be effective at taking care of both yourself and the other person.

Assertive communication, while especially designed to alter the misbehavior, is also a great way to set the stage for discussion about the pain or mis-education. In contrast to angry outbursts, martyr-like acceptance or emotional withdrawal, assertive communication is a direct, non-attacking and indeed caring approach to problem solving. As such it makes it easier for the other person to listen non-defensively, and to open up with regard to what is going on from his or her point of view.

The four basic steps for assertive communication are surprisingly simple. You say something like:

1. "When you do X (the misbehavior),
2. "I feel Y (an unpleasant emotion),
3. "I don't like to feel Y. One possible solution that might serve us both would be that you do Z instead of X, and
4. "How do you feel about that?"

The crucial elements of each step are also simple and straight-forward:

1. *When you do X . . . .* Here you introduce the problem, describing the misbehavior and situation in specific, factual terms. Betty introduces the problem well when she says to Maurice, in a relatively conversational tone,

"You said that you would watch the kids while I jogged. When I returned, I found a pitcher of spilled milk on the kitchen floor, the kids eating frosted cereal on our living room rug, and you in your study, working on a business report."

Betty could have introduced the problem using judgmental or emotionally loaded phrases, such as "neglecting the kids"; she could have attacked his personality, perhaps with something about "indulging in your workaholism"; and she could have suggested bad motivations on his part, maybe saying "you don't care about us." Also, she could have implied such things by using an angry or strident or whiny tone. Saying or implying any of these things might have felt satisfying for a moment, whether or not she was accurate. Unfortunately, such words or tone would have invited defensive quibbling, defensive counter-attack, defensive derailing from the main topic, or defensive withdrawal on Maurice's part. As it was, her simple, factual statement was hard to argue with, and it made it easier for him to listen to what follows:

2. *I feel Y.* Here, the key concern is to express your feeling without suggesting some bad motive on the other person's part. Betty does this well when she says to Maurice,

"When something like this happens, I don't feel safe to go off and jog."

Betty avoided making dark accusations about Maurice's motives, such as, "I feel like I've been had!" or "I feel like you are trying to keep me fat!" Most people don't like being accused of bad motives, and even if Maurice indeed has bad motives, he is unlikely to admit them while under attack.

Sometimes the other person will respond to the "I feel" statement with something like, "It's silly for you to feel that way!" To prevent that sort of comment from derailing you, briefly say something like, "Look, whether it seems silly or illogical or different from the way you would feel, I'm telling you it's the way I feel."

If this doesn't stop the person, and he/she persists in a sort of "I'm-gonna-have-the-last-word" game, short-circuit such a contest by saying, "Well, perhaps we'll have to agree to disagree on that, but here's the main point: (and move on to #3).

3.   *I don't like to feel Y. One possible solution that might work for us both would be that you do Z instead of X.* Here, the key is for you to say what you want changed (to not feel Y), that you know of a solution that would work for you (doing Z instead of X), and that you are open to other good solutions that might come up in this discussion (yours is a possible solution but not necessarily the only good one). Betty does this well when she says, "Fitness is really important to me, but I've got to feel safe to do it. One possible solution would be that I'll give you any protection you need from interruptions to work on your reports, but when you're taking care of the kids, you'll have that be the only thing you're doing."

Here, Betty is inviting Maurice to take her concerns seriously, she doesn't assume that her solution has to be THE solution, and she recognizes that Maurice probably has a concern, too. None of this is likely to be a threat that Maurice has to defend himself against.

4.   *How do you feel about that?* Actually this may be the most important sentence of all. It gives special emphasis to the fact that rather than attacking the other person, you want to have a two-sided, problem-solving discussion. Up until now, you've had the floor. The discussion has been one-sided. Now it's time to listen. Although the person doing the misbehavior was inconsiderate of your needs, you are trying to encourage a considerate approach on both sides. So, sticking with our example, Betty says,

"How do you feel about that?"

At this point, Maurice may come up with a variety of responses. If he feels supportive of Betty's jogging and has only lapsed into momentary workaholism, he may simply apologize, agree with her proposed solution, and then help clean up the messes in the kitchen and living room. On the other hand, if he actually has qualms about her getting fit, or if he is feeling overwhelmed by his work, or if he never knows what to do around little kids, or if having to watch kids is totally different from what he grew up to expect, or whatever his concern, maybe he'll start talking about it when she says, "How do you feel about that?" If he does, Betty and Maurice very likely will need more than one discussion to get things worked out, but they've got a start. That start is important and it might not have happened if Betty had aggressively taken the offensive or had simply said nothing.

Using process comments.
Assertive communication increases the chances of a win-win solution, but does not guarantee it. Depending on the circumstances and the other person, your attempts at it may or may not be appropriate. If you decide that a win-win solution is not possible, I still would encourage you to take care of yourself while causing as little harm as possible to others, including to the one doing the misbehavior. Sometimes you can do this with what psychologists call process comments.

Rafael, a colleague of mine, provided an example of process comments when he (somewhat) politely got rid of a door-to-door salesman: Initially, Rafael made hints that the salesman should leave, but the salesman ignored these and instead kept asking questions. Sometimes he used what Rafael answered as new lead-ins to keep the conversation going.

Finally, Rafael said, "You know, I've been trying to tell you in nice ways that I don't want your products and that I don't want to continue this conversation, but you keep coming back with more things. That's not being respectful of me and it annoys me. Now I'm going to say 'good-bye' nicely, and I hope you'll do the same. Either way, though, I will next close the door.

"Now, good-bye; have a good day."

The salesman said, "Good-bye," with a somewhat surprised look on his face, and Rafael closed the door.

Process comments like Rafael's focus less on the content of the other person's communication and more on the communication's pattern and its negative impact on you. In some cases, the other person doesn't intend to have this negative impact and will be glad to stop doing the misbehavior, once you give him/her your clear feedback. In other cases, the bad intention is there, and your process comment exposes his/her "game." Once exposed, any further occurrences of it won't come off quite so innocently.

Here are some fitness-related examples:

Becky to her mother-in-law: "Mom, I'm sure you mean it as a joke, but when you ask me who I'm slimming down for, it makes me feel as if you don't have a very high opinion of me or my commitment to your son. That doesn't feel very good."

Ann to her next-door neighbor Howard: "Howard, I know you mean to be friendly, but your jokes and compliments about my appearance, my exercise and my fitness level make me feel uncomfortable and make me want to avoid having any contact with you. Please stop."

Josh to Jim, his sometimes drinking-buddy who sulks when Josh says he's going to work out, rather than going drinking with Jim after work: "Hey Jim, why the long face and the droopy shoulders? You look as if I'm rejecting you as a person when I tell you I'm going to work out instead of going drinking with you. That feels unfair. Are you rejecting me if you refuse my invitation to go with me to the gym? Come on, man!"

As with assertive communication, process comments like these describe the misbehavior in factual, non-attacking terms that are hard to quibble with. Process comments include an "I feel" message and at least a semblance of civility. In contrast to assertive responses, however, they don't make an attempt at mutual problem solving and they only consider one remedy. Whether implied or stated explicitly, your process comment asks the other person to "please stop" the unwanted behavior. Also, you don't offer an opportunity to explore the other person's needs or concerns. Finally, in contrast to the "win-win" outcomes that assertive responses aim at, process comments more readily settle for "win-lose" outcomes, with the one commenting being the "winner." Ideally, however, you as commenter will not stomp the "loser" into the ground and ideally (if desired) you will remain able to maintain your relationship with him or her.

Saying the right things to yourself.
Whether you respond assertively, make process comments, or follow a less structured approach, you will be more effective if you operate from a positive foundation. As with many things, what you say to yourself can be at least as important as what you say to others. Self-statements like the following contribute to a positive foundation:

> "I have the right to follow a fitness lifestyle, and am not a bad person for trying to do so."

> "I am trying to find a reasonable approach to that lifestyle."

> "The fact that this other person has pains or mis-learnings does not make me a bad person for seeking a reasonable approach."

> "The other person isn't a bad person either. Demonizing solves nothing. My empathy may help us solve our problem."

Grounding yourself in concepts such as these will help you be more relaxed, less threatened, and thus less threaten*ing* as you approach the other person. With such grounding, you can articulate more patiently what you want to do and why. If appropriate, you can invite the other person's participation. Whether the other person does or does not choose to participate, you can more easily request support or at least non-interference from him or her. If it fits, point out how the other person might also benefit from your progress. In particular, your calm, clear efforts may provide enough assurance and encourage enough openness to enable the other person to discuss whatever pain your fitness activity is triggering. If you can learn what that pain is and if you can make an empathetic connection with it, the other person will have less reason to want to fight you and more reason to want to jointly work things out. All of this flows most easily from the constructive things you have told yourself.

Springboard.

1. *Get grounded.* Before you try assertive communication or process comments, make sure you are grounded. Your ability to achieve your goals is greatly enhanced when you can articulate to yourself where you stand and are comfortable with that stance. Perhaps start by re-reading the self-statements in the preceding section. Know

how you feel about these ideas. The people who are putting up the social obstacles may disagree with them, and they may be well practiced in presenting contrary views. Before talking with them, think the ideas through, perhaps airing them with a neutral friend.

2. *Get clear.* After you are grounded, consider several more steps before actually confronting the offending person. Whether you choose the assertive approach or the process comment approach, think through what you want to say. Make what you say be consistent with your grounding.

3. *Practice.* Mentally rehearse how you might say your concerns under several different possible situations. Better yet, role-play some likely scenarios with your neutral friend. Sometimes, as you do this, have your friend play the offender's role while you confront assertively or make process comments. Other times, switch roles. Along with having what you say be consistent with your grounding, also practice having how you say it be consistent with your grounding. That is, have your tone, posture, facial expression and word choices be those of a relaxed, confident person, one who wants a change to occur, but preferably in a way that leaves everybody whole. Finally, when possible, keep it simple, and don't be afraid to repeat yourself (calmly).

This can be fun, especially the role playing, and you and the friend you practice with will probably enjoy a few laughs in the process. Most importantly, though, you'll lose some of the inappropriate inhibition that most of us feel when first trying to do this. Ultimately, practice is the key. You'll get better at effectively expressing your concerns as you go along.

4. *Don't give up prematurely.* Of course, when you actually try your new approach with the offending person, the real life scenario will never be exactly the way you planned it. That difference may be enough to throw you off. You may fail or you may not even try—that time. Don't be discouraged. Instead, retreat, take your time, think through (possibly again with your friend) how you might have handled things differently, and then get ready for next time. The more you learn from these experiences, the more prepared you'll be for the offending person's next surprise. And there might be more surprises. In their pain and as a result of their mis-learnings, some offenders have developed fairly large repertoires.

5. *Keep grounded.* Before, during, and after any assertive or process confrontation, stay focused on your grounding. Generate security from the fact that you are asking for something both reasonable and legitimate. Reduce any misplaced

guilt you may feel by making sure you approach the offender from an attitude of good will. And regardless of the outcome—even if the offender remains steadfastly dedicated to placing obstacles in your path, and even if you have to consider less desirable approaches—comfort yourself with the knowledge that you tried to improve matters in a mature, civilized way.

INTERNAL OBSTACLES

The Problem: Seeing the big picture accurately.

IF YOU HAVE "the big picture" of a fitness lifestyle in mind, a picture with good information on things like costs, benefits, expectations of success, and plans, you'll more easily achieve good motivation and good follow through. Unfortunately, your own internal obstacles may make it hard for you to see that picture accurately. Current emotional feelings, physical feelings or drug/alcohol induced states can alter your perceptions of facts. Your values, attitudes and coping skills can further alter those perceptions. Equally problematic, some internal obstacles can keep you from even seeing all of the facts, accurately perceived or not. In this chapter, I will identify several common internal obstacles, some well known, some not, and suggest ways you can overcome them, maintain motivation, and follow a fitness lifestyle.

SOLUTIONS

Addressing drug/alcohol issues.

Once I worked with a musician who aspired to be a concert soloist. His problem was that he couldn't make himself practice. That is, he found it very hard to initiate or persevere when working on difficult musical passages. He would justify his retreats from practice with reasons he'd later acknowledge to be pseudo-intellectual rationalizations. During our assessment, he confided that he smoked pot each evening with a fellow musician. When I suggested that smoking pot might affect his motivation and practice, he said that his friend had no similar difficulties. I then pointed out that people vary greatly, and that instead of comparing himself to his friend, he should compare himself to himself—himself under "pot-free" conditions versus himself under "pot-altered" conditions. Each morning for the next several weeks, he kept track of how his music practicing went, with some mornings preceded by pot use the night before, and others not. He found that on mornings after smoking pot the night before, he continued to have poor motivation and ineffective practicing. On mornings following "clean" evenings, he had excellent motivation and effective practice sessions. As a result of his self-evaluation, his friend lost a smoking buddy.

While pot and alcohol are perhaps the most common chemical detriments to good motivation, they aren't the only ones. Depending on the drug and your dependency level, you may not be able to cut back safely and/or effectively without medical supervision, so please check with your physician.

Addressing emotional problems.
Exercise can contribute to person's emotional well-being. However, certain emotional conditions, most notably depression, can severely undermine motivation.[22] If the benefits of exercise seem trivial to you, if the costs seem unduly huge, and if (to your friends) your expectations for success seem unduly pessimistic, begin by getting a physical exam, for possible physical problems as well as for depression. Depending on the outcome of that, you may want a referral to a licensed and reputable psychiatrist, psychologist or social worker. Among the attributes of a reputable mental health professional should be his or her open mindedness to the use of counseling and/or to the use of medications, depending on what you, the individual patient, need.

Addressing "hang-ups."
There is a joke about a pastor who urged one of his elderly parishioners to think more about the "hereafter." In response, the parishioner, with a twinkle in his eye, said, "I think about the hereafter all the time. I'm always going around my house, from one room to another, asking myself, 'Now what am I here after?'" Unfortunately, whether in a joke or in reality, a declining memory is

not the only internal obstacle that can cause you to lose track of what you are "here after," including when you're pursuing a fitness lifestyle. I call some of these obstacles "hang-ups." They are ways of handling things like values, attitudes and fears that—while not necessarily pathological—can still cause you or me to sometimes forget what we are "here after" and fail to achieve our goals.

Rebel hang-ups. Harry provides an example of what might be called a "rebel hang-up." Harry was in his late thirties when he joined a Tae Kwon Do club at a local university. His goals were to learn self defense, increase his flexibility, and keep in shape. The club was known for its physical rigor and its authoritarian approach. Also its members, mostly college students, were known for their high levels of proficiency, morale and camaraderie. They met three times each week, for 90 minutes each time.

From the start, the sessions were demanding. The instructors cut little slack for beginners, having them work as hard as everyone else. As a result, the club had a high initial dropout rate. Harry anticipated this, and got into fairly good shape before joining. Thus, beyond a few aches and pains during the first couple of weeks, he handled the rigor part just fine. In fact, he liked it. He also liked the emphasis on good technique.

What he didn't like was the club's strict, authoritarian discipline. If he was late to class, he immediately had to drop to the floor and do 20 push-ups. If he forgot and wore his wristwatch to class, he had to do 20 more push-ups. If he wasn't paying attention and messed up a drill, he had to do yet 20 more push-ups. Since he was in good shape, he didn't mind the push-ups, but he hated the idea of having to "take this stuff" from the instructors who were all at least 15 years younger than he was. Once when he really messed up, an instructor had him face the rest of the club members who then shouted in unison, "You suck!" Worst of all (for him), he always had to say, "Yes, sir" or "No, sir" when addressed by his youthful instructors.

When others were similarly disciplined, they took it in good humor and recognized it as part of what helped the club function so well. Harry reacted differently. Despite the obvious rewards of getting in better condition, becoming more flexible and getting increasingly proficient in Tai Kwon Do, he came home more and more angry as the sessions went on. Finally, toward the end of practice one day, in response to an instructor's correction of his jump-spin-crescent kick, Harry hissed, "Shove it, SIR!" and stormed out of class. He never went back.

Prior to joining the club, if Harry had been asked whether it was more important to have the benefits of the Tae Kwon Do club or to avoid the club's discipline, he would have said the benefits were more important. That would have been his rational side speaking. His rational side would have said, "I won't let this authoritarian nonsense cheat me out of the benefits."

Unfortunately, as the classes went along, Harry's emotional side took over, leading him to recall old hatreds of conformity, and reenact confusions between being a rebel and being an individual. Individuals keep their goals in mind and work toward them, whether that requires temporary conformity, temporary rebellion, or finding new paths. Rebels want to be individuals too, of course, but mistakenly feel that to be individuals they must resist the authoritarian and fight back. Unfortunately, resistance and fighting back doesn't always get them to their goals. To be individuals, as well as to achieve their goals, rebels need to have their rational sides ask their emotional sides, "What am I here after?"

Rebellion doesn't only happen in Tae Kwon Do clubs. For example, have you ever "rebelled" against the diet your nutritionist prescribed or against the exercise program your personal trainer gave you? In your "individual" mode, if you had difficulties with the program, you probably would have talked things over with the nutritionist or trainer, and mutually sought a goal-related alternative, rather than passively or actively resisting the prescription.

Competitive hang-ups. Rebel hang-ups aren't the only way that maladaptive values, attitudes, coping skills and misconceptions can congeal into internal obstacles and get any of us off-track. For example, do you ever get overly competitive with yourself, emotionally putting your ego on the line when you exercise?

Dave and Lola went on a mountain hike. They thought this would be a relaxing way to exercise on Sunday afternoon. Part way up the mountain, Dave got locked into the idea of going all the way to the top. With considerable effort, they eventually got there. Unfortunately, by the time they did the sun was setting and they had to go all the way back down in the dark, stumbling along, cold, overly fatigued and sometimes losing the path. Lola, realizing that this was how some hikers got seriously injured, was terrified.

Certainly no one would say Dave was a "quitter." But that's not what he was "here after." Dave and Lola went on the hike to have some relaxing exercise, not to prove that Dave was not a quitter. As it was, by just getting cold and tired, Dave got off relatively easyily. He could have gained an injury—or lost a girlfriend.

Status quo hang-ups. [23] Some people, ostensibly wishing to design fitness programs for themselves, spend a lot of time and energy without ever embarking on a program. If this could be you, ask yourself whether your progress toward exercise seems to stay stuck at the talking level. Are you always seeking additional information or telling anyone who will listen about your past efforts or entering into philosophical discourse about this or that approach—but never doing anything to change your *status quo?* Do all of the conditions have to be just right before you are ready to give fitness a fair try? Do you, ignoring the truth in what Voltaire said about the perfect being the enemy of the good, require some sort of guarantee that everything will work perfectly before you take "the leap?"

If so, maybe it is time to look inside yourself, not outside, to identify the obstacle causing you to maintain the *status quo*. Very likely, fear will be a big component—maybe fear of risking failure, fear of self-ridicule, or fear of being out of your comfort zone. Try to identify your fear. Then make it come out into the open by writing down its themes, patterns and impacts. Make the fear known. Known fears are easier to confront, overcome or work around. One caution, though: please don't let this internal search become yet another delaying tactic! Start your fitness program (knowing that you can change details as you progress) and also start looking inward. Let the two processes help each other and help you move from the *status quo*.

Spontaneity hang-ups. Spontaneity gives us some of the "spice" in our lives. What a drag if we had to justify and plan everything we did. Sometimes on a weekend afternoon, for example, if the weather is nice, it's fun to say, "Hey, let's throw some food together, grab a Frisbee, and have a picnic in the park!" Who wants to have to analyze things first, exploring questions like, "Now let's see... what happened the last time we had a picnic? Are you sure the good weather is going to last? Shouldn't we talk this over first?" There are good reasons why we like to be spontaneous part of the time.

On the other hand, spontaneity can go too far. A picnic with no plates or utensils—not so much fun. Some things, including a fitness program, happen best with a reasonable amount of analysis, planning and routine. In certain ways, the world belongs to those who plan. Few good programs get started, and even fewer get continued, by people who drift about like dry leaves, blown here and there by the winds of impulse and chance.

In a way, spontaneity hang-ups—insisting on too much spontaneity—can have much of the same impact as *status quo* hang-ups: in both cases, the changes you hope to make don't happen enough. Often, these two hang-ups have something else in common: fear. Of course, if you lead an overly spontaneous life, some of your chaos may be due to outside factors; but consider stepping back for a moment and looking inwardly, too. Your chaos may be helping you dodge some fear. In the long run, you'll be better off facing the fear and finding constructive ways to overcome it.

Addressing pessimistic perceptual habits.
Think of your perceptual habits, the ways you view the world around you, as your tendencies to see—or not see—certain things in your life. One boss may see creativity in a suggestion you make, while another may see discontent or competition. Which boss will you give your next suggestion to? One teacher may tend to see spunkiness and intelligence in your child's high activity level,

while another may see misbehavior. Which teacher will you prefer to trust your child to? Whether a person's perceptual habits developed from positive or negative past experiences, the perceptual habits definitely affect what the person sees and how he or she will act.

Two basic perceptual habits can especially undermine your motivation for a fitness lifestyle. Both of these habits are forms of pessimism, and both will interfere with your ability to see "the big picture."

Seeing the glass half-empty. This habit is so well known in other contexts that it has long been a cliché in our culture. Other people can teach you to see the glass half-empty instead of half-full without necessarily intending to.

That's what Jethro taught his team. Jethro was a high school football coach. As with any high school team, his players were not fully mature, whether physically, emotionally, or in terms of football skills and savvy. While many of them showed flashes of potential, all provided Jethro with plenty of examples of deficits that he roundly criticized. Long ago, Jethro's mentor had told him, "Make those kids mad enough, and they'll work their butts off to prove you wrong!"

The players did get mad. Unfortunately, most of them also developed doubts about their abilities to succeed, many came to see the costs of playing football as exceeding the benefits, some quit, and the remainder only worked hard when under Jethro's steely gaze.

At the end of another losing season, Jethro shared his woes with a friend. He blamed the team's losses on the players, on their "coddling" parents, and on a "soft work ethic" throughout the school. It didn't occur to Jethro that he had played a significant role.

Thanks to Jethro's coaching approach, his players developed the perceptual tendency to see the glass half empty instead of half full. In effect, they came to wear pessimistic blinders that caused them to see only their current deficits. A better trained coach would have taught them to see "the big picture." That picture would include not only the deficits but also the potentials that the players could fulfill with hard work. Also a better coach would have instilled the idea of gradual improvement and he/she would have celebrated the players' progress with them, rather than only criticizing their remaining deficits. With this approach, the players would have had more motivation, they would have worked harder, and they undoubtedly would have improved. Be your own best possible coach!

Over-emphasizing recent negative experiences. All of us have times when the glass doesn't have to be even half empty for us to focus on the pessimistic version. Have you ever had a week where six days were great, but on the seventh day a lot of things went badly? Imagine that at the end of that bad day someone asked you how your week was. If you answered, "Except for today, it's been great," you'd be looking at the "big picture." If you instead answered, "Terrible," you over-emphasized the most recent day's negative experiences. Perhaps in your mind you only saw that day's problems and totally missed all the rest of the week. Perhaps you undervalued what had happened on the six good days, given the bad day.

If you follow this tendency with your fitness efforts, it can wreak havoc with your motivation. After all, one basis for your expectations of future success is your (undistorted) memories of past successes. Your sense of daily benefits, as well as costs, relies heavily on your accurate memory of past experiences as well as your feelings about them. If the positive memories are blocked out or trivialized by today's setbacks, the viability of your motivation will be very tenuous.

That's what happened to Sandy: Sandy was a thirty-five-year-old modern dance teacher. She was also a heavy smoker, having started in her mid-teens. Over the years she had made some brief attempts to stop smoking, but always started up again when she was under stress or had gained a few pounds (a bad way to control weight!). The only times she was able to break the smoking habit were during her two pregnancies. Each time, though, as soon as she was able to, she was smoking again.

Sandy regularly danced with her pupils, and until recently that activity plus her smoking had kept her quite trim. Unfortunately, following her second pregnancy, this approach no longer worked. Not only did she find herself keeping the extra weight from the pregnancy, but she realized she was slowly gaining more weight. On top of this, her husband, Cliff, increasingly urged her to stop smoking.

Hoping to finally succeed, Sandy set up a combined smoking cessation and running program. Her plan had her start running at a gentle level, gradually increasing her weekly mileage while gradually decreasing her daily cigarette consumption. She was good at keeping other calorie-related activities constant, like her diet and her dancing, and somewhere during the first five weeks of this program, she found herself losing weight.

On the eighth week, she had several setbacks. First, her weight loss hit its first plateau. Then her children got sick, keeping her and Cliff up most of the next couple of nights. Between her children's extra needs and her dance classes, she couldn't run for most of the week. Meanwhile, as she dragged through each day, she tried to perk herself up by snacking and by smoking more. At the end of the week, when she finally ran again, she tried to over-compensate for the week's extra caloric build-up by running faster and further than she was ready for. As a result, she severely aggravated an old dance injury in her left foot. She realized she would neither be able to dance nor run for at least the next three weeks.

In frustration, she told Cliff that the running was incompatible with all the demands on her and didn't seem to help that much anyway. Besides that, she said, she didn't see the need to stop smoking. After all, her grandmother, who was eighty-six, "has smoked all her life and is doing fine."

For Sandy, the tendency to over-emphasize recent bad experiences had developed long before these incidents. Fortunately, she soon recognized that, and decided to make a change. Here's what happened: When this sort of thing had happened in the past, Cliff had tried to talk Sandy out of her distorted perspective. He found that to be a pretty futile and punishing exercise. This time, he simply said, "Well, it's your decision." Then he picked up a children's book and began to read to their four-year-old daughter. His response caught Sandy off-balance. She realized that she had expected him to criticize her decision, just as he had in the past. With no one to justify herself to, she realized she'd followed this pattern too often. Perhaps she needed to try something new.

Later, she described her change: "Imagine being in a room where looking at most of the things in it make you feel 'good.' Now, along with these 'good' things, there is also a sheet of red paper that represents a problem, and looking only at it can make you feel 'bad.' If you can see all the things in the room, both the 'good' things and the red paper, you of course know that you have a problem to deal with (whatever the red paper represents), but the 'good' outweighs the 'bad,' and basically you feel OK. Next, imagine that the red paper somehow gets right in front of your eyes, blocking out the view of all the 'good' things. All you see is red, and you feel terrible—maybe so terrible that you don't feel like doing anything. Next, imagine putting the paper at arm's length, so you can still see it, but now you can see all the 'good' things too. When you put the paper at arm's length you can relax enough to deal with your problem. The paper doesn't change in size, but now it hits you less hard.

"I needed to get the red paper at arm's length so I could take both it and the good things seriously. I mean to say at arm's length emotionally. To get things at arm's length, emotionally, I first grabbed another children's book and read to our two-year old. Then, after the children went to bed I cooked a special asparagus soup that Cliff's grandma used to make.

"I waited until the next morning to figure out what to do about my program. I decided that while the children were still getting well, I would focus on catching up on my sleep, on cutting back on cigarettes again, and on just doing stretch exercises with my dance students. Then, after the children were well and I had more time, I got an aqua-jog belt and did deep water running while my foot was still injured. Finally, when my foot recovered enough—and that took a full month—I gradually worked into dancing with my students and then into running too."

Usually the perceptual habit won't go away immediately. It will come back again when other problems come up. But the habit weakens each time you stop the perception when you realize it has started. As soon as you realize you are over-emphasizing a recent bad experience, begin applying the steps listed below. Initially you may not realize you are into the maladaptive pattern until you're already pretty discouraged. Over time you'll catch yourself earlier in the pattern and be able to stop the process more quickly. Eventually, your tendency to over-emphasize recent setbacks will fade away. Here are the steps:

1. Acknowledge your pain. Acknowledge that today's problem isn't designed to feel good. It is going to feel bad, and pretending that it's trivial runs the risk of making you feel like a weakling, since it still hurts. Also, acknowledge that right now you are not in the right emotional state to appreciate the good things that have been going on. That will come later.

2. Seek relief and perspective. Because the problem isn't trivial, you need relief. Getting relief isn't escapism. You'll be coming back to the problem, but you'll come back better prepared. "Relief" isn't being like an ostrich with its head in the sand, either. Rather, like Sandy's example, it's putting the problem at "arm's length" to regain the big picture. Different people do this in different ways—one person might do something physical like taking a hot bath or a jog, while another might immerse himself or herself in a novel for a couple hours.

Many people do not succeed when they try to get relief and perspective with alcohol. It's a depressant, despite any initial buzz, and it can further distort your perception of the problem. Watching TV or browsing the internet for hours may not be very helpful either, particularly if the content is vacuous enough to leave lots of opportunity for the "red paper" to pop back in front of you.

3. Evaluate your alternatives. After you've gotten the problem at arm's length, examine the alternatives your problem suggests, including the alternative of quitting your fitness program. Also, re-examine your fitness program. Each alternative has some benefits and some costs. Of course, I'm hoping you won't like the cost/benefits ratio you'd get from totally stopping your program. On the other hand, the "problem" may prove to be a helpful "flag," telling you that you need to at least modify your program a bit.

4. Make a choice on what you want to do with your fitness program and plan accordingly.

5. Celebrate. Celebrate whatever you've learned from having undergone the problem. Celebrate the fact that you countered this pessimistic perceptual habit, or that you figured out a better approach, or that you'll have prevented future setbacks.

6. Re-adjust your expectations of fitness progress to be in keeping with whatever changes you've chosen.

Springboard.

The first step in reducing or eliminating an internal obstacle is to recognize it as a problem. Unfortunately, none of us tend to be very objective when looking at our internal obstacles. We think the distorted pictures of reality that our obstacles cause are . . . well . . . reality. Try these three questions to help increase your objectivity:

1. If I saw someone else doing what I do, would I think his or her motivational problem might be related to an internal obstacle?
2. Would my motivational difficulties make more sense if this alleged obstacle was indeed interfering with me?
3. Do I have anything to lose by exploring this possibility further?

If your answer to the first two questions is "yes" and your answer to the third is "no," I'm hoping you will make use of the ideas in this chapter.

AFTERWORD

Control and Choice

I've written the *Guide* with the assumption that we're all able to exert some control over our lives. Note the word "some." Used here, the word "some" has very different consequences than the alternative words, "no" or "total."

If you assume that you have no control of your life, you'll probably sink into passivity—like why bother? On the other hand, if you assume you have total control, you may try to exert total control and doom yourself to frustration, since no one actually has total control. Then, like many before you, you also may give up and sink into passivity. I hope that at least with regard to exercise and fitness, you'll embrace the assumption of some control, that you'll figure out the extent of that control, and that you'll choose to exert control within that range.

Best wishes.

ENDNOTES

Foreword

1. See Centers for Disease Control and Prevention (2015). Quoting from the overview of this document:

Regular physical activity is one of the most important things you can do for your health. It can help:

- *Control your weight*
- *Reduce your risk of cardiovascular disease*
- *Reduce your risk for type 2 diabetes and metabolic syndrome*
- *Reduce your risk of some cancers*
- *Strengthen your bones and muscles'*
- *Improve your mental health and mood*
- *Improve your ability to do daily activities and prevent falls, if you're an older adult*
- *Increase your chances of living longer*

Chapter 1

2. See Liberman (2005) and Schultheiss, et.al. (2012) for encyclopedic summaries of the general field of motivation.

3. See reviews by Gollwitzer (1993; 1999) and Rhodes & de Bruijn (2013).

4. See Kiernan, et. al (2013).

Chapter 2

5. See Endnote 1 again for some possible ideas.

Chapter 3

6. See Bandura (1997) and Warner, et. al. (2014).

7. Armitage (2005) suggests that a person needs to be following an exercise program for at least five weeks before doing so becomes a stable habit.

Chapter 4

8. I am indebted to the work of Ryan and Deci (2000) for their research and theorizing concerning intrinsic motivation and integrated extrinsic motivation. My emphases on validation, ownership and mastery come from their work.

9. See Higgins (1997).

Chapter 5

10. See Lakein (1973).

11. See Covey (1989).

12. I am indebted to Roberts and Treasure (1997) for my discussion on "ego vs task orientation."

13. See Csikszentmihalyi (1999).

Chapter 6

14. This section derives from "Implementation Intentions" research in the psychological literature. While adhering to the key concepts from this research, I have altered some of the terms with the hope of increasing accessibility and applicability to a lay readership. The Implementation Intentions approach was introduced and developed by Gollwitzer (1993; 1999).

Chapter 7

15. See Schneider (2001).

Chapter 8

16. Again see Endnote 8.

17. Again see Endnotes 10 and 11.

Chapter 9

18. Fear of potential harm from exercise has been observed by researchers studying the elderly and disabled, including Lundgren (1980), Resnick, et. al. (2006), and Tierney, et. al. (2011).

19. See Office of Disease Prevention and Health Promotion (2015). This document provides updated information on the CDC 2008 Physical Activity Guidelines, along with other helpful exercise-relevant information.

I encourage you to seek personalized, professional guidance, but this information can prepare you to ask better questions as you consult.

20. Obviousuly I endorse the notion of exercising with other people and the benefits they can offer you. My only caveat would be that you not have your exercise be so dependent on others that your program disintegrates if those other people become temporarily or permanently unavailable.

Chapter 10
21. I am indebted to Jacubowski and Lange's (1978) book for my discussion on assertive communication.

Chapter 11
22. See Kangas, et. al (2015).

23. I am indebted to Kulh's (1984) concept of "state orientation" for my discussions of both "*status quo* hang-ups" and "spontaneity hang-ups."

WORKS CITED IN ENDNOTES

Armitage, C.J. (2005). Can the theory of planned behavior predict the maintenance of physical activity? *Health Psychology 24 (3), 235-245.* doi: 10.1037/0278-6133. 24.3.235

Bandura, A. (1997). *Self-efficacy: The exercise of control.* New York, NY: Freeman.

Centers for Disease Control and Prevention (2015). *Physical activity for everyone: The benefits of physical activity.* Retrieved from http://www.cdc.gov/physicalactivity/ basics/pa-health

Covey, S,R, (1989). *The 7 habits of highly successful people.* New York, NY: Free Press.

Csikszentmihalyi, M. (1999). If we are so rich, why aren't we happy? *American Psychologist, 154,* 821-827.

Gollwitzer, P.M. (1993). Goal achievement: The role of intentions. In W. Stroebe & M. Hewstone (Eds.), *European review of social psychology, 4* (pp. 141-185). Chichester, UK: John Wiley & Sons.

Gollwitzer, P.M. (1999). Implementation intentions: Strong effects of simple plans. *American Psychologist 54 (7),* 493-503.

Higgens, E.T. (1997). Beyond pleasure and pain. *American Psychologist 52 (12)*, 1280-1300.

Iso-Ahola, S.E. (2013). Exercise: Why it is a challenge for both the nonconscious and conscious mind. *Review of General Psychology 17 (1)*, 93-110. Doi: 10.1037/a0030657

Jacubowski, P. & Lange, A.L. (1978). *The assertive option.* Champaign, IL: Research Press.

Kangas, J.L., Baldwin, A.S., Rosenfield, D., Smits, J.A., Jasper, A. & Rethorst, C.D. (2015). Examining the moderating effect of depressive symptoms on the relation between exercise and self-efficacy during the initiation of regular exercise. *Health Psychogy 34*, 556-565. doi: 10.1037/hea0000142

Kiernan, M, Brown, S.D., Schoffman, D.E., Lee, K., King, A.C., Taylor, C.B., Schleicher, N.C. & Perri, M.G. (2013). Promoting healthy weight with "stability skills first": A randomized trial. *Journal of Consulting and Clinical Psychology 81 (2)*, 336-346. doi: 10.1037/a0030554

Kuhl, J. (1984). Volitional aspects of achievement motivation and learned helplessness: Toward a comprehensive theory of action control. In B.A. Maher &

W.A. Maher (Eds.), *Progress in experimental personality research,* (pp. 99-171). New York, NY: Academic Press.

Lakein, A. (1973). *How to get control of your time and your life.* New York, NY: New American Library.

Liberman, N. (2005). Motivation. In L. Nadel (Ed.) *Encyclopedia of cognitive science 3* (pp. 103-111). Chichester, UK: John Wiley & Sons.

Lundgren, H.M. (1980). Motivation for participation in adult fitness programs. In G.A. Stull (Ed.) *Encyclopedia of physical education, fitness and sports 2* (pp. 525-530. Salt Lack City, UT: Brighton.

Office of Disease Prevention and Health Promotion (2015). *Physical activity guidelines for Americans.* Retrieved from http://www.health.gov/paguidelines/guidelines/summary.aspx

Resnick, B., Vogel, A. & Luisi, D. (2006). Motivating minority older adults to exercise. *Cultural Diversity and Ethnic Minority Psychology 12 (1),* 17-29. doi: 10.1037/1099-9809.12.1.17

Rhodes, R.E. & de Bruijn, G.J. (2013). How big is the physical activity intention-behaviour gap? A meta-analysis using the action control framework. *British*

Joural of Health Psychology 18 (2), 296-309. doi: 10.111/ bjhp.12032

Roberts, G.C. & Treasure, D.C. (1997). Motivation in physical activity contexts: An achievement goal perspective. In M.L. Maehr (Ed.) *Advances in motivation and achievement 10* (pp. 413-447). Bingley, UK: Emerald Group.

Ryan, R.M. & Deci, E.L. (2000). Self-determination theory and the facilitation of intrinsic motivation, social development, and well-being. *American Psychologist 55 (1)*, 68-78. doi: 10.1037//0003-066X.55.1.68

Schneider, S.L. (2001). In search of realistic optimism: Meaning, knowledge, and warm fuzziness. *American Psychologist 56 (3)*, 250-263. doi: 10:1037//0003-066X. 56.3.250

Schultheiss, O.C., Strasser, A., Rosch, A.G., Kordik, A. & Graham, S.C.C. (2012). Motivation. In V.S. Ramachandran (Ed.) *Encyclopedia of human behavior, second edition 2* (pp. 650-656). San Diego, CA: Academic Press.

Tierney, S. Mamas, M., Skelton, D., Woods, S., Rutter, M.K., Gibson, M., Neyses, L. & Deaton, C. (2011). What can we learn from patients with heart failure about exercise adherence? A systematic review of qualitative papers. *Health Psychology 30 (4)*, 401-410. doi: 10:1037/a0022848

Warner, L.M., Schuz, B., Wolff, J.K., Parschau, L., Wurm, S. & Scharzer, R. (2014). Sources of self-efficacy for physical activity. *Health Psychology 33 (11)*, 1298-1308. Doi: 10:1037/hea0000085

9 781983 938351